(JOHN GOEUROT)

THE REGIMENT OF LIFE, ADDED A TREATISE OF THE PESTILENCE, THE BOOKE OF CHILDREN

LONDON, 1546

WALTER J. JOHNSON, INC.
THEATRUM ORBIS TERRARUM, LTD.
AMSTERDAM 1976 NORWOOD, N.J.

The publishers acknowledge their gratitude to
the Curators of the Bodleian Library, Oxford,
for their permission to reproduce the Library's
copy, Shelfmark: 8°.P.24 Med.

S.T.C. No 11969

Collation: a^8, A-X^8, Aa-Cc^8

Published in 1976 by

Theatrum Orbis Terrarum, Ltd.
Keizersgracht 526, Amsterdam

&

Walter J. Johnson, Inc.
355 Chestnut Street
Norwood, New Jersey
07648

ISBN 90 221·0802 3

Printed in the Netherlands

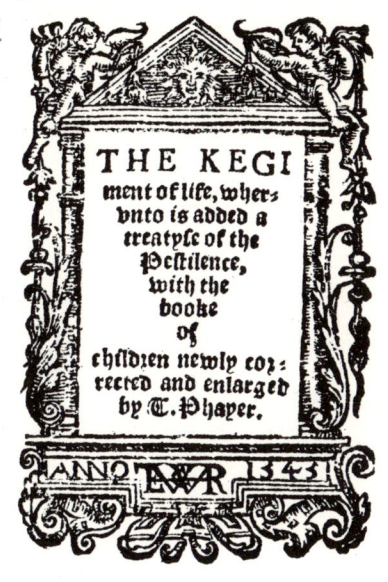

THE KEGI
ment of life, wher=
vnto is added a
treatyse of the
Pestilence,
with the
booke
of
children newly cor=
rected and enlarged
by T. Phayer.

ANNO 1543.

The preface to the boke of children.

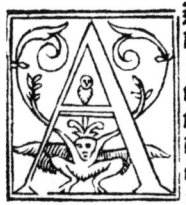

Althoughe (as I doubt not) euerye good man wil enterpret this work to none other ende but to be for the comforte of them that are diseased, and will esteme no lesse, of me by whom they profyte, then they wyl be glad to receyue the benefites: Yet forasmoche as it is impossible to auoyd the teeth of malicious enuye, I thought it not vnnecessary to preuent ÿ furyes of some, which are euer gnawynge and bytynge vpō them that further any godlye sciences. To those I protest that in all my studyes, I neuer entended,

nor

A preface

nor yet do entẽd to satiffy the mindes of any such pikfaultes (which wyll do nothynge but detract and iudge other, snuffynge at all that offendeth the noses of theyr mompshe affections, howsoeuer laudable it be otherwayes) but my purpose is here to do them good that haue moost nede, that is to say chyldren, and to shewe the remedyes that god hath created for the vse of mã, to distribute in Englissh to them that are vnlerned part of the treasure that is in other lãguages, to prouoke them that are of better lerning, to vtter theyr knowlege in suche lyke attemptes, finallye to declare that to the vse of many, whiche ought not to be secrete for lucre of a fewe, and to communicat the frute of my labours, to them that will gently and thankefully

to the reader.

fully recepue them, whiche yf any be so proude or supercilious, that they immediatly will despise, I shall frendly desyre thē, wyth the wordes of Horace Quod si meliora nouisti, Candidus imparti, si nō his vtere mecum. If they know better, let vs haue parte: yf they do not, why repine they at me, why condempne they the thinge that they cannot amende? or yf they can, why dissimule they theyr connynge? how longe wolde they haue the people ignoraunt? why grutche they phisike to come forth in Englysshe? wolde they haue no man to knowe but onely they? Or what make they thē selues? Marchauntes of our lyues and deathes that we shulde bye our healthe onely of them, and at theyr prices? no good phisicion is of that mynde.

For

A preface

For yf Galene the prynce of thys arte beinge a Grecian wrote in the Greke, king Auicenne of Arabie in the spech of his Arbyans: Yf Plinius, Celsus, Serenus and other of the Latines wrote to the people in the Latyne tōge, Marsilius Ficinus (whome all men assente to be singulerly learned) disdayned not to wryte in the language of Italy: generally, yf the entent of all that euer set forth any noble studye, haue ben to be redde, of as many as wolde. What reason is it that we shuld huther muther here amōge a fewe, the thyng that was made to be common vnto all. Chryst sayeth, no man lyghteth a candle to couer it with a bushell, but setteth it to serue euery mans nede: & these go about, not only to couer it when it is lyghted, but to

quēch

to the reader.

quench it afore it be kidled (if thy myght by malyce) whyche as it is a detestable thynge in any godlye science: so me thynketh in thys so necessarye an arte, it is excedynge dampnable and deuylyshe, to debarre the fruycion of so inestimable benefytes, which our heauenlye father hath prepared for oure cōfort & innumerable vses, wherwyth he hath armed oure impotent nature agaynst the assaultes of so manye sycknesses: wherby his infynyte mercye and aboundaunte goodnesse is in nothynge els more apparauntly cōfessed, by the whiche benefites, as it wer w moost sensible argumentes spoken out of heuen, he constraineth vs to thinke vpon our owne weakenes, and to knowledge, that in al flesh is nothynge but myserie, siknesse, sorowes,

A preface

sorowes, synne, affliction, and deathe, no not so moche strengthe as by our owne power, to relyeue one member of our bodyes diseased. As for the knoweledge of medicines, comfort of herbes, mayntenaunce of healthe, prosperytie, & life, they be hys benefyttes, and procede of hym, to the ende that we shulde in common, helpe one an other, and so lyue togyther in hys lawes and commaundementes: in the which doyng we shall declare oure selues, to haue woorthelye employed them, and as frutefull seruauntes, be liberallye rewarded, Otherwyse, vndoutedly the talente whyche we haue hydden shall be dygged vp, and distributed to them that shall be more diligent, a terrible confusion afore so hye a iustyce, & at suche a court where

to the reader.

where no wager of lawe shall be taken, no proctoure lymytted to defende the cause, none exception allowed to reproue the wytnes, no councell admytted to qualifye the gloses, the very bare texte shalbe there alleged. Cur non posuisti talentum in tenus. Why haste thou not bestowed my talēte to the vantage. These and suche other examples, haue enforced me beynge oftentymes excercysed in the studye of phisike, to deryue out of the purest fountaynes of the same facultye, suche holsome remedyes, as are most approued to the consolation of them that are afflycted, as farre as God hathe gyuen me vnderstanding to perceyue: folowing therein, not onlye the famous and excellent authours of antiquitye, but also the mē of hyghe learnyng nowe

A preface

now of oure dayes, as Manardus, Fuchsius, Ruellius, Musa, Campegius, Sebastyan of Austryke, Otho Brunfelsius, Leonellus. &c. wyth dyuers other for myne oportunitye, not omyttynge also the good and sure experimentes that are founde profitable by the daylye practyse.

And where as in the regiment of lyfe, whyche I translated out of y freuche tonge, it hath appered to some, more curyouse than nedeth, by reason of the straunge ingrediens, wherof it often treateth: Ye shal knowe that I haue in manye places amplyfyed the same, wyth suche common thynges, as may be easelye gotten, to satysfie the myndes of them that were offended, or els cōsiderig that there is no moneye so precious as helth,

to the reader.

I wold thinke no spice to dere, for mayntenauns therof. Notwytstandynge I hope to see the tyme, whā the nature of Simples (whyche haue ben hytherto incrediblie corrupted) shal be redde in Englysche as in other languages, that is to saye the perfecte declaration of the qualities of herbes, seedes, rootes trees, and of all commodities that are here amongest vs, shalb earnestely and trulye declared, in oure owne natyue speche, by the grace of god. To the whyche I trust allerned men (hauynge a zele to the common wealth) wyll apply theyr diligent industries, surely for my parte, I shall neuer cease, during my breath, to bestowe my labour

A preface.
to the furtheraunce of it (tylle it
come to passe) euen to the
vttermoste of my sim=
ple power. Thus
fare ye well
gentle re
ders.
∴

⸿ Londini, Mense. Junij.
1.5.4.6.

387355

WILLIAM F. MAAG LIBRARY
YOUNGSTOWN STATE UNIVERSITY

¶ Here beginneth the Regiment of lyfe, and first of the nature of mannes bodye.

☙ The humours whyche be in nature and howe they are deuyded.

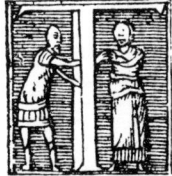

He bodye of man is compact of foure humours, þ is to saye: Bloud, Phlegme, Choler, and Melancholye, whyche humours are called the sonnes of the Elementes, because they be complexioned lyke the foure elementes. For lyke as the ayre is hote and moyste: so is the bloud hote and moyest. And as fyer is hote and drye: so is choler hote & drye. And as water is colde and moyst: so is phlegme colde and moyste. And as the yearth is colde and drye: so melancholy is colde and drye. Whereby it apereth

A   that

The regiment

that thre be nyne complexions. Wherof .iiii. be symple, that is to wete hote, colde, moyst, and drye, and .iiii. cõplexions compounde: that is, hote and moyst, whych is the complexion of the ayre and of blood. Hote & dry, whic is the complexion of the fyre, and of cholere. Colde and moyst, which is the cõplexion of the water and of phlegme and colde and drye, that is the complexion of earth and of melancholye. The nynth complexion is temperate, neyther to hote nor to colde, nor to moyste nor to drye, whych yet is a thyng very seldome sene amonge men. After the phisicions, the sayde foure humours gouerne and rule euery one in his place and enduce men to be of the complexions folowynge.

❡ The complexion of the phlegmatyke.

Phlegme

of lyfe. fol. ɛ

Phlegme enclyneth a man to be
- well formed.
- a sleper.
- dull of vnderstandyng.
- full of spattle.
- full of coloure.

¶ The cōplexions of the sanguyne.

Blood causeth one to be.
- full of flesh.
- liberall.
- amyable.
- curtyse.
- mery.
- inuentyue.
- bolde.
- lecherous.
- of red coloure.

¶ The cōplexions of the cholerike.

Cholre causeth a mā to be
- hastye.
- enuyous.
- couetous.
- subtyle.
- cruell.
- a watcher.
- prodigall.
- leane, and of yelowe coloure.

A.ii.   The

The Regiment

⁋ The complexions of the melancholyke.

Melancholye maketh one,
: Solitarye.
Soft spirited.
Fearfull.
Heauye.
Curyous.
Enuyous.
Couctous.
Blacke of coloure.

⁋ These be the foure humours wherof the bodyes are cōpounded, and euery one of them hath a special dominiō in respect of all the other, accordyng to the age, that is to saye, from a mānes natiuitie, tyl he come to .xxv. yeres, the bloud hath most power, and from that tyme to the yeare of his age .xxxv. raygneth the Cholere, for then commeth heate into the vaynes, and the cholere begynneth to aryse and be strong.

Then cōmeth myddle age, and bryngeth for the melancholye, an humoure colde and drye and hath his enduraūce

tyll

The Regiment of lyfe.

tyl fyfty yeres or therabout, at whiche tyme all the humours of the bodye begynne to dimynysshe, and the natural heate by lytle and lytle doth abate. And then succedeth olde age vnto deth in the whiche age phlegme hath ÿ principal power and dominion. Wherfore it shalbe necessary for al that be of that age to côfort their bodyes with some natural heate and meates of good norysshynge, as yolkes of egges potched good and yonge flesshe, wheate bread, & good wyne, and all suche thynges as engendre good bloud and spirites, wherof we entende (by the sufferaunce of God) to declare more aboundauntlye hereafter.

¶ Here followeth the description of inwarde and outwarde diseases, with the most holsome and expert remedyes for the cure therof, appropriate to euery membre thoroughout the body.

A.iii.   The

The regyment

⸿ The fyrst chapter, of the syckenesse and remedyes of the heed.

HEad ache chaunceth often tymes, of dyuers and sondry causes as of bloud, cholere, fleume, or melancholye, or of ventositie, and somtymes of heate of the sunne, or of to great colde of the ayre.

Ye maye knowe head ache when it commeth of bloude, for in the face and eyes there appeareth a darke rednesse, pryckyng and heuynesse with heate.

⸿ Remedye.

Ye must let hym bloude on the hed veyne, on that syde that the peine is on then laye vpon the place oyle of roses, vynegre, and rosewater, or a bag wyth roses spryncled with rosewater. And here is to be noted, as wel in this cause as all other, that if his bellye be harde and bounde, fyrst ye must gyue hym an easye glyster, or els halfe an ounce of Cassia newlye drawen out of the cane, or some other easye laxatyue to pro=
uoke

uoke the dutye of the wombe, els all applications of medicynes, wyll be nothyng worth at all.

One may knowe head ache that proceedeth of cholere, when in the face there is a clere rednesse, enclynyng somwhat toward yelowe, holownesse of the eies and the mouth drye and hote: And sometymes bytternesse, small reste, greate heate with sharpe payne, chefely on the ryght syde of the head.

¶ Remedye.

Ye must gyue hym morne and euen to drynke, sirupe of vpolettes, or pome granades with a meane draught of endyue water in a glasse, or of comyn water sodden and cooled agayne. And in steade of these sirupes ye maye drynke water of endyue, succorye, purcelane, & nenuphar mengled togyther, or one of them by them selfe, two or iii. dayes at euenyng and mornyng. Then gyue a dramme of pillule sine quibus, at night to bed warde, or about mydnight, & the day folowing kepe you in your chãber.

The Regiment

In stede of those pylles it is good euery mornig to take an houre afore sūne a medicine to drynke, that shalbe made of halfe an ounce of Succo rosarum, mixt with two ounces of water of endyue. In stede of the sayde succo rosarum, ye maye take halfe an ounce of diapruinis laxatiue, & ye muste take hede in gyuyng suche purgacions, that the pacient be strong, for if he be weake, ye may gyue hym but the halfe of ỹ sayd pylles or of the other laxatyues. And yf in diminyshyng the quantitie of the sayde medicines, it worketh not wyth the pacient as it shulde, it is conuenièt to gyue hym a common glister.

¶ An other remedy for the
same peyne.

Ye must laye theron a lynnen cloth moysted in rosewater, plantayne water, morel water, and vynegre, or elles take the iuyce of lettuce and roses, and a litle vyneger, and warme it together and dyppe therin a lynnen clothe, and laye it to the peyne.

of lyfe. fol. v
An other.

Ye muſt take the whytes of .ii. egges wyth roſe water, and beate it well togyther: and wyth towe or flaxe: laye it to the greued place. Also ye muſt ſhaue his heed, and mylke thereon womans mylke, that nouryſheth a wenche, or waſſhe hys heed with warme water, wherin haue bene ſodden vyne leaues, ſage, floures of water lilies, and roſes Alſo it is neceſſary to waſh his feete & legges wyth the ſayde watter, ſo that the pacient haue no reume: for yf there be reumatike matters, ye ought nether to ſhaue his heed, waſh his legges, nor to laye any colde thyng or moyſt to hys heed. Ye maye knowe that fleume is cauſe of the peyne in the heed, when ye fele coldneſſe with great heuyneſſe: ſpecyallye in the hyndre parte: when one ſpytteth often, and hath hys face lyke ſunne brent.

¶ Remedye.

Ye muſt drynke .iii. or iiii. mornynges ſirupe of ſticados with water of fenell

The regiment

or sirupe of wormewood, with a decoction of sauge and maioram. Then ye muste pourge the head from the sayde fleume, with pillule cochie, and wyth pylles of agarici, or pillule auree made wyth one of the sayde syrupes, fyue in a dramme, and take. iiii. or. v. at nyghte to bedwardes, or about mydnight. Or in stede of those pylles ye maye take a potion i the morninge. v. houres afore meat, made of halfe an ounce of diacartami dissolued in. ii. or. iii. ounces of betonye. After that ye ought to comforte the heed, by wering of a copse, made of double lynnen cloth, and sowed lyke a cotten quylte, wherin ye must put floures of camomyl, maioriim, cloues, nutmygges, maces, graynes of Paradyse and cynamome in pouder, for suche thinges digest the fleume, so that a purgation be gruen of the sayde pylles, or of pylles assagareth or pylles of hiera picra, which are not so laxatyue as the other are,

After the sayde purgation, ye muste put

of lyfe.　　Fo. vi.

put in the nose of the pacient, pouder of pellitorie of Spayne or other, to make him to nese. Also it is good to gargarise his mouth, with water wherein sage hath ben sodden, and then to annoynte his heed with oyle of lilyes, camomill or of rue.

Beside this, it is good to gyue the paciēte euerye mornynge to drynke, sage wyne w̄ water, to consum: y̆ fleume and to comfort the brayne and the sinowes. The sayd wyne is thus made.

Put a lytle bagge ful of good sage bruised in a quart of newe wyne, & let it stande so a nyghte, then wringe it out, & vse it. Suche wyne of sage the inhabiters of Parysc & Fraunce vse to drynke after harueste al the wynter longe.

When peyne of the head procedeth of melancholic, the paciēt feleth heuines of the heed, & hath terrible dreames, w̄ great care & thought, or feare, and hys peyne is specyally vpon the lefte syde.

⸿ Remedye.

Take

The regyment

Take sirupe of borage, hartes tongue or fumytorye, with water of buglosse: and hartestonge, or with the decoction of sage or tyme, for by these sirupes ye shall digest and correct the sayd melancholyke humours, and within a whyle the peyne wyll be released. And yf it cease not for these medicines, after ye haue vsed .ii. or iii. dayes one of ye sayd sirupes, or two or thre of them togither take a dramme of pylles, halfe auree: and halfe sine quibus, or elles halfe of hiera, and alfe of pilles of fumitorie, or in stede of pylles, ye maye take in the mornyng fyue houres afore meate .iii. drammes and an halfe of diasene, tempered in water of borage or hoppes, or in the decoction of sage, licorice, greate reysins, and cordial floures & frutes

Heed ache cometh of wynde or ventositie, whē the pacient thynketh that he heareth sounde or noyse in his heed, & the peyne is flytteryng from on place to an other, wythout heuynesse or descendyng humoure,

Re-

Remedye.

Lay vnto his heed hote lynen clothes and make a bagge of Gromell seedes, & baye salte dryed togyther in a panne: so procede wyth stronger thynges, yf nede require, as is bagges made of ma iorym, rosemarye, rue, barberies, & iuniper beries, laide to þ payned place or with the decoction of the foresayde thynges, make fomentation or embrocation vpon his heed.

In other remedye.

Ye must take oyle of Camomyll, oyle of Dyll or Lylies, & annoynte the hed wyth one of them, or wyth, ii, or, iii, or all togyther. Yf that helpe not, take oyle of Rue, Spike, & of Castor, & anoynt it therwyth: and adde therto a lytle Pepper, and mustard seede, yf ye wolde haue it sore chafed or hette. Also it is good to drawe vp by the nose, water of Honye, þ iuyce of Maiorim, & of Fenel, aromatised with & Nutmyg ge & lignum aloes.

Rasis a great practicioner amonge phisicions

The regyment

phisitions sayth, þ whosoeuer often tymes putteth into hys nose the iuyce of maiorim, shall neuer be diseased in þ heed. I thynke he meaneth of the great maiorym.

Yff peyne of the heed come of heate of the sunne, ye muste applye to the places diseased, as it is sayde in the remedyes of cholere.

But yf the sayde payne procede of coldenesse of the ayre, then vse as it is sayde afore in the remedyes of fleume.

¶ Here foloweth a regiment agaynst all diseases of the heed

The patient that is diseased i þ hed, whether it be of bloode, or of cholere, may not drike wyne nor eat mochflesh whit meates nor thynges that gyue any great nouryshement. But must be contented to drinke ptisane, barly water, or iulep of roses, & to eate rosted apples, damaske prunes, almon mylke, hulled barlye, and pottage made with lettuse, sorell purce-

purcelane, in brothe of peason, or with a chycken, or veale, yf the pacyente be feble.

When payne procedeth of a colde humour, the paciēt oughte to drynke no wyne in thre of the fyrst dayes, but to drynke onely penyale, or suche smalle drynke, for although the wyne be very comfortable, as cōcernyng naturall heate, yet it is contrarye and hurtefull vnto the spirites animal of the braine, and also of the sinnowes.

And the paciētc oughte what payne soeuer it be of the head, to forbeare all vaporous meates, as garlike, onions, lekes, pease, beanes, nuttes, mylke meates, spyces, mustarde, great colewoortes, salt meates, and meates of yll dygestion. Also he muste abstayne from slepe of the daye, and after supper by the space of two houres.

Trauayle of the mynde is very cōtrary, bycause of the cōmotiō that happeneth vnto þ lyuely spirites, which are instrumētes of vnderstādīng, as suice
that

¶e regyment

that noble phisicion sayeth, i the chapiter de soda tempoꝛali. Nihil est adeo conueniēs sode tempoꝛali, sicut tranquillitas τ dimissio totius quod commouet sicut sūt foꝛtes cogitatiões. ꝛc. There is nothyng that is so cōuenient foꝛ the meygrym, as tranquillitie and rest, and let al thinges passe that moue the vertue animal, as great musynges and all laboure of the spyꝛites. And chefely one ought after dinner to kepe hym from all thynges that trouble the memoꝛye, as studyinge, reedynge, wrytyng, and other lyke.

And foꝛ the better vnderstandyng of the syckenesse chaunsyng in the heed, ye shall knowe, that somtyme it chaunceth bicause of other diseased mēbꝛes as of the stomache, oꝛ of the mother of the reines, of the liuer, oꝛ of the splene and not of any cause in the heed it self. Therfoꝛe ye ought to cure soche sycknesse by helpyng of the same mēbꝛes, as it shalbe shewed i the chapiters folowynge.

And

of lyfe.   Fol. ix.

And ye maye knowe, that the heade ache cometh of diseases of ye stomake, when the paciēt hath greate payne at the stomake. Of the mother, when the woman feleth greate payne in her bellye. Of the reynes when their is a great payne in the backe. Of the splene, whē he feleth payne & heuynesse therabout, vnder the lyft syde. Of the lyuer, whē the payne is in the ryght syde, aboute the lyuer which is beneth the rybbes.

¶ Remedies appropriate to the head of what cause soeuer the payne be.

Take an handfull of Betony, an handfull of Camomylle, and a handful of veruayne leaues pickled, stampe them and seeth them in blacke worte, or in ale for lake of it, and in the latter ende of the seethynge, put to it a litle Comyn brayed, the pouder of a hartes horne, & the yolkes of two egges, and safrō a lytle, stirre thē wel about and lye a playster hote ouer all hys forehead and temples. This is an excellent remedye also for the mey-
        B.   gryme.

gryme. It shall perce the better yf ye adde a lytle vinegre.

¶ Another.

Make a plaister of bean floure lineseed & oyle of Camomylle, or in lacke of it goose grece or duckes grece, and rubbe the place with Aqua vite, and after lay the playster hote vpon it.

¶ An other.

Take a sponeful of mustardeseed & another of Bay buryes, make them in pouder and stampe them with a handful of earthe wormes, splitte and skraped from their earth, and a litle oyle of Roses, or of Camomyll, or capons grece and lay it on the grefe.

Also it is good to take y̆ iuce of Iuie leaues mixte wyth oyle, and vinegre, & to rubbe therwyth your temples, and your nosethrilles.

Also the Chestwormes that are found betwene the barkes of trees, whiche wyl turne them selues togyther lyke a beade when they be touched yf they be taken & sodden in oyle it maketh a singuler of lyfe. Fol. x.

guler oyntment for the meygryme.

℃ The seconde chapter, how to cure diseases chauncyng in the face.

Yrst as touchynge a disease called Gutta rosacea, or copperface in englysh, it is an excessyue rednes about þ nose, or other places of the face, commynge of brent humours, or of salte phlegme, whych can not be holpen, yf it be rooted and olde.

℃ Remedye for the same yf it be curable.

Ye must giue him a purgacion, as is said ĩ þ payne of þ head, commyng of choldre, thẽ dyppe lynnẽ clothes in alume water, whyche shal be made thus. Take a poũde of alumeglasse, þ iuce of pureclanc, of plãtayne, & vergiouce of grape or crabbes, of eche a pint & a halfe with þ whytes of .xx. egges & beate thẽ well togyther with þ said iuce, thẽ mixte al togyther and distylle it in a cõmune stillatorie, & kepe the water for to vse agaynste all

B.ii. pym=

pymples, scurfes, wheales, chafinges, and heates that chaūce in the skynne. The clothes dipt as is aforesaid, must be layed to the rednesse, and oftētymes renewed wyth other freshe cloutes dypped in the same.

⁋ Another remedy.

Take lytarge of sylver, and brymstone, of eche lyke muche, and seeth thē in rose water and vinegre, & then with a lynnen cloute wette in the said vinegre, lap it to the sore.

⁋ Remedye to pallisye the coppred face that is uncurable.

Make a bath wyth the floures of camomyll, violettes, roses, and floures of water lyllyes, thē annoynt the place with unguentum album cāphoratum, and mixt that ointment wyth a lytle yelowe brymstone, and quycksyluer kylled wyth fastyng spytle, and annoynt the place wythal.

⁋ A water for the same.

A water called lac virginis, is very good, & rosewater mixt with sulphur, oyle

oyle of tartare, and oyle of wheate. Also these thinges are good for tetters, & other ruggednesse of the skynne. The sayd lac virginis claryfyeth the face, & dryeth vp moyste pymples, and taketh awaye freckels of the vysage, & is thus made. Take .iii. ouces of literge of siluer fine poudred, halfe a pinte of good whyte vinegre, mixt them togyther, & distylle them by a fyltre, or throughe a lytle bagge or by a pece of cloth. Then take of the same water, and myngle it wyth water of salte, made wyth one ounce of salte poudred, & halfe a poūd of rayne water, or wel water, and mingle these waters togyther, and it wyll be whyte lyke mylke, and wyth thys rubbe the corrupt place. Some adde a lytle ceruse wyth the lytarge whych is good for all rednesse of the face.

Here foloweth a general diete for al copperous faces.

ABstayne from all salte thynges, spices, fried meates, and rosted meates. Also from drynking of wyne,

The Regyment

for it is verye euyll. Also onyons, mu=
ſtarde, & garlycke, are verye nought.
In ſtede of whiche ye muſt take pur=
cellane, ſorel, lettuce, hoppes, & borage,
with ſuccory or endyue, i potrige or o=
therwiſe. Alſo it is neceſſarye to be la=
xatiue, & i ſlepig, to laye your head hye.

For rednesse of the face that is not coppeꝛoſed.

Take a pynt of goates mylke, the
cromes of one whyte loſe hote, the
whyte of ſyxe egges, canfere two dꝛa=
mes, and the iuyce of ſyxe cytrons,
mixte all theſe togyther wyth the ſayd
mylke, then take all the thꝛe kindes of
plantayne, and put them in the ſtylle
vnder the ſayde dꝛugges, and after it
an other bedde of the ſame. iii. ſoꝛtes
of plantayne, and diſtylle them wyth
an eaſy fyre as ye wolde diſtylle roſe=
water, and kepe it in a glaſſe veſſel.
And after. xv. daies take a white lyn=
nen cloth, and dyppe in the ſaid water
and laye it to the redneſſe.

And other for the ſame.

Water

of lyps. fol. xii.

¶ Water of lylyes styllcd, wyth the bloode of an oxe, and a lítle camphere, is very good.

¶ For chapped or skabbye lyppes.

¶ Innoynt them wyth vnguentū album cāphoratum, and yf there be any corrupt blood, or matter, ye must wash the place wyth water of Plantayne, wherein hath bene sodde a litle a lume afore ye put on the sayd oyntment.

¶ For the same.

¶ Unguentum de tutia and oyle of yolkes of egges, be verye good for it. Also it is good to wash ye place wt plātayne water, & barlye water togither.

¶ For cankers, vlcers, and
Noli me tangere.

Forasmuch as Noli me tangere chaunceth often in the nose or aboute the face, begynnynge of a lytle harde and round kyrnel, or knobbe, and ful of payne, declyning towarde a pale and leady colour, ye maye iuge that diseafe verye peryllous, notwithstādig it is good to anoynt

B.iiii.

The regym ent.

noynt it as hereafter foloweth, and also to applye therto other remedyes, as this.

℣ Take Unguentum album two or thre ounces, the iuce of plantayne and nightshade, of eche halfe an ounce Tutie the weyght of halfe a crowne, mingle them togyther, and make an oyntment whyche is good for ẏ same disease.

℣ For wormes in the face.

Although that wormes in the face maye not be had out, but wyth great difficultie: and by lõge processe, bycause of the colde humour whereof they come, neuertheles, forasmuch as oftentymes they happen vnto poore folkes, here shall be recited a receypte proued for the same disease, whyche is an oyntmente of a singuler operatiõ: and is thus made.

℣ Take the leaues, ⁊ rootes of lekes, ⁊ iuce them al togyther, and take therof a pynt and a halfe, ⁊ put it ĩ a glasse with an ounce of pouder of pellitorye,
and

of lyfe. Fol.xiii.

and a scruple of verdegrece, and stirre them all togyther, and euery day bathe the sayde wormes and wheles, wyth rotten moysted in the said iuce, & stirre it often in the glasse, thys is good also for wormes in any other mēbres, and bredynge in the sychenesse called in Fraunce the kynges euyl.

¶ A purgation whiche ye ought to take before the said bathynge.

¶ Take halfe a dramme of good turbyth, and a scruple of gynger, halfe an ounce of suger, & a lytle whyte wine, mixte all togyther, and drynke it in the mornynge twyse a weeke warme, and renewe it euery thre wekes.

¶ For an vlcered face through wormes.

Ye muste fyrste mundifie the deade flesshe wyth Unguentum egyptiacum, or the pouder called precipitatus, and for the perfecte curacion ye must drye it well, wherfore it is good to wasshe the place often with alume water, and put therein lynte, and yf there be great

moystnes

The Regyment

moystnes at the time of desiccation, ye must dyppe the same lynte in vnguentum apostoloru̅ or ceraseos, with a lytle of the oyntment y̅ foloweth, which ye maye safely applie from the begynning to the ende of the cure, for it hath vertue to clense and incarnate, wyth a gentle mundification an dryer.g.

⁋ A singuler oyntment for wormes that matter.

Take oyle of lyllyes, oyle of lynseed, ana. ounces. iii. oyle of roses, oyle of myrtylles, ana. ounces. ii. lytarge of golde and sylver, and redde leade, ana. i. ounce, diaquilon whyte wyth gummes, iiii. ounces, goates tallowe, hogges grece, of eche two ounces & a halfe, blacke pytche, and colophonye, of eche ii. ounces, of the iuyce of hou̅deslonge, iiii. ounces. Seeth al togyther tyl they be blacke and the iuyce be cleane consumed then streyne it thorow a thycke canuase, and after seeth it agayne til it be excedyng blacke in colour, and then adde to it cleare turpe̅tyne, iii. ounces,

gume

of lyfe.　　　Fol. xliii.

gum: oppoponax, ii. ounces & an halfe, white waxe as muche as shal suffice to make a plaister not ouer hard, & put ye turpentine & oppoponax i̅, whē ye take it frō the fyer. This is an excellēt playster also both for woundes & vlcers.

For the same.

It is very good to lay vpō the ye herbe called houndstōg stāped wt a litle hony.

¶ Regyment or diete for the same sicknes.

¶ The paciēt in al diseases of ye face must endure hunger as muche as is possible, and eate not muche at once. Also he muste holde his head vpryghte, and slepe not on his knees nor elbowes, nor wyth hys face bowed downe. Also he must forbeare muche laughynge, speakynge, and great anger.

¶ For the eyes.

Hereafter foloweth diuers medicines for the eyes, whyche are the wyndowes of the mynde, for both ioye & anger, and the moost of our affectiōs, are seene & knowen openlye through them,

them, and they are ordeyned and made to lighten al the bodye, where vnto nature hathe gyuen browes and eye lyddes, to defende them and kepe them in safetye, and the better to resist thiges contrary and hurtfull vnto them.

Yet notwythstandyng, besyde many other chaunces, there happeneth sõtymes a debilitye in the syght, whiche must be holpen as hereafter foloweth

☞ Take fenell, veruepne, celydone, rue, eyebryght, and roses, of euerye one of them a lyke muche, and distylle them as ye wolde distille rose water, and vse a lytle therof in youre yes, bothe i the mornynge, & when ye go to bedde.

☞ A water proued to clarifye the
 dymnes of the syght.

☞ Take the iuyce of fenell, of celydonye, rue and eyebryght, of eche .ii. ounces, honye an ounce and a halfe, aloes, tutye, and sarcocolle, of eche halfe an ounce, the galle of a capon, chcken or cocke two drammes, nutmygges, cloues, and safron, of eche a dramme, suger

get candy.vi.drammes, put al in a lembike of glasse & distille it. And of this water put in your eyes onces i the day And if ye coulde gette the liuer of a he goate, and mixt wyth the said thinges in the distyllation, the water wyl be of muche greater vertue, & almost without comparison.

⁋ For the same.

Ye must vse euerye daye to eate nutmygges, and to take onces in a weke I mirabolane condyte.

⁋ For the same.

⁋ Take a pye and burne her, & beat her to pouder, and mingle it wyth fenel water, and put it in your eyes. Also water of younge pyes styled, is verye good. Lykewise water of rotten apples put, ii. or. iii. droppes i the eyes helpeth very muche.

A singuler water for diseases
in the eyes and to clari-
fye the syght.

Take the grene walnuttes, huskes and al, from the tre with a feawe walnut

The Regyment

nut leaues and diſtylle therof a water to droppe wythin your eyes.

Pylles good for the ſyght.

The pylles ſine quibus, aſſagareth, with troſciſkes of agaryk, and pillule lucis, are excellente good to purge the brayne and comfort the ſyght.

For payne of the eyes.

Somtymes payne of the eyes commeth of bloud, and then the vaynes of the eyes are redde and ſwollen, wherfore it is conueniēt to be let bloude of the heade veyne on the ſyde where the payne is.

For bloodeſhoten eyes.

The bloode of a ſtockedoue or in lacke of it an other doue or pigeō dropped a lytle in the eye and a wete cloute thereof layde vpon the ſame, healethe bloodſhoten eyes whether it be of ſtroke or any other cauſe.

Somtime the ſayd peyne cōmeth of cholere, & then the patient feleth great heate ſharpe prycking, & much peyne, & commonly there appeareth no gumme

in the

of lyfe.   Fo.xvi.

in the eyes, and yf it do, it is yelowe. Therfore ye ought to gyue hym a purgatiō purgynge cholere, as hath bene sayde in the remedye of the head proceedyng of the cause of cholere.

⁋ For swellynge of the eyes.

Take a quynce and seeth it in water tyl it be softe, then pare it & bruse it & mixe it wt the yolke of an egge & the cromes of wheaten or white bread steped in ye said water & put therto a litle womans milke and two peny weyght of saffron, brape them al togyther and laye it ouer the forehead and the eyes.

⁋ Sometymes suche paynes chaunce bycause of fleume, and then the paciēt feleth great heuynes in his eyes, with abundaunce of gummy matter, or water descendynge into the eyes. And in thys case, ye muste purge the fleume, as it hathe bene sayde in the remedye of the heade greued by the excesse of fleume.

⁋ To resolue the gumme ye shal vse to washe your eyes often tymes wyth
the

the iuyce of housleke otherwyse called sengreene.

¶ And some tymes the same peyne cōmeth bycause of ventositye or wynde, and then the pacient feleth suche peynes as if one beate on his eare with an hammer, for which it is good to make a decoction of camomille floures, melliloce, & fenel seed, in water and whyte wyne & therin wette a foure double linen cloth & the licour wel pressed out, laye it often vpon the eye.

Otherwhyles there chaũseth peyne of the eyes bicause of exterior thinges as of wynde, duste, or heate of the sōne and then it is mete to laye therto womans mylke, well beaten with the whyte of an egge.

And sometyme the sayde peyne commeth by percussion or strykynge, and then ye muste droppe into the eye, of ȳ bloud of a pigeons wynge, or of a partryche, whyche bloud hath lyke vertue to take awaye spottes, markes, and rednes of the eyes.

For

For very great payne of the eyes.

Take an ounce and a halfe of oyle of roses, the yolke of an egge, & a quarter of an ounce of barly floure, and a lytle saffron, myxe all togyther & put it betwene .ii. lynnen clothes, and laye it to the peyne.

And other.

Take of cromes of wheaten breade whyte, an ounce, and seeth it in nyght shade or morell water, then myxe with the said bread .ii. yolkes of egges, oyle of roses, and camomil, of eche an ounce and an halfe muscilage of lineseede an ounce, and use it as is aforesayde.

An other.

Take syxe leaues of henbane, & rost them, then beate them verye well in a morter, and laye them to the peyne.

For rednes of the eyes.

In the begynnyng of the rednes lay vpon the eyes towe dypped in the whyte of egges, but let the whites be wel beaten fyrst wyth rosewater, or with plātayne

The Regyment

tayne water.

¶ An other.

Take redde roses, and seeth them and let them be set warme to your eye This taketh away spottes of bloode, that somtyme chaunceth in the eyes.

Also it is good for all diseases of the eyes. And it is good for rednes of the eyes, that commeth by stryking or any such vyolence. If at any time ther happē a spot or blemish iṅ ẏ eye, by a stroke ye muste laye to it by and by, towe wet in rosewater and in whytes of egges, and after that the peine be mitigate ye must lay a playstre vpon the eye, made of a rawe egge, barlye floure, and the iuyce or muscilage, of mallowes, and then yf the eye be not holpen of ẏ sait bloud, ye must laye to it a plaster both dissolutiue, defensiue, and partlye appeysynge the peyne, whyche muste be made of whete floure, the iuyce of mallowes, mintes, and smalache, and the yolke of an egge.

¶ Of hardenesse that hath ben
longe

of lyfe.   fol. xviii.
longe in the eye.

¶ Take a scruple of aloes succotrine & melte it in water of celydony at ye fyre then receyue the fume of it, and afterwarde wash the eye with fenel water.

¶ An other.

¶ Take poudre of cumyne mytt wyth waxe lyke a playstre, and laye it vppon the eye.

¶ An other.

¶ Take red roses, sage, rue, celedonie of eche a lyke moche, wyth a lytle salte and distil a water, and putte thereof a drop or two in your eye, euenynge and mornynge. In steade of that water, it is good to take iuyce of verueine, rue, and a lytle rosewater.

¶ For all rednesse of the eyes.

¶ Take the bygnesse of a nut of white copperose, and a scruple of peros, and poudre it, and mixte it with a glassful of well water, then putte two or thre droppes in your eyes.

¶ For the same,
L.ii.   Wates

The Regyment.

Water of strawburies made and put in the eye is good.

¶ A singuler poudre that dryeth and taketh away rednesse of the eyes.

Take tutie preparate an ouce, antimonie halfe an ounce, perles two drammes, red coral a dram, and an halfe, pouldre all these thynges verye fyne, & kepe them in a boxe of tynne, and use it.

¶ For to stoppe wateryng of the eyes.

Make a plaister of poudre of mastike, fyne frankensence, boole armoniake, and gume dragagante, with whytes of egges myxte togyther, & layde to the foreheade & teples. Also it is good to set ventoses on the nape of the necke. Also it is good to make a colirse to put into the eyes, as foloweth. Take tutie preparate and the stone called lapis hematites, of eche a dramme, aloes halfe a drame

of lyfe. Fol.xix.
a dramme, perles and camphore, of eche a scruple, poudre them all verye fyne, and myxe them in the iuces of water distilled of the knoppes of rooses, and therof make a colliric.

Also for to stoppe al humoures descendynge to the eyes, these thynges aforesayde are verye good myxte with rayne water, wherin olibanum or frankensens hath bene sodden.

¶ For webbes of the eye.

It maye be easelye holpen in yong folkes, but in aged persons it is very harde. And in the begynnynge ye must mollifye them wyth a decoction of the floures of camomyl, mellilote, and cole leaues, receyuyng the fume of the sayd decoction wythin the eyes, and then put therin a lytle poudre made wyth sugre candie, sall gemme, and egges shelles burnt, and afterwarde distil into them womans mylke wyth the decoction of fenugreke.

¶ An other singuler receat for

L.iii. webbes

The Regyment
webbes in the eyes.

Take snayles wyth the shelles on, and wash them eyght tymes, and distil them in a common styllatorye, than take hares galles, redde corall, and sugre candye, wyth the sayde water, distylle them agayne, and put euery mornyng and euenyng a drop in your eye.

¶ An other water.

This water is made of whyte coperose suger candy, and rosewater, with whites of egges that are sodden hard, all streyned through a lynen cloth, and put into youre eye, after dyner and at nyght to bedwarde.

¶ Regiment for them that haue any sore eyes.

Ye must alway kepe your belly lose and abstayne from fyre, smoke, wynde dust, and ouer hote or colde ayer, & from weppynge, and longe reading of a smal letter, from ouer longe watchyng, ouer moche drinkynge of wyne, and eatyng late, for al these are very noysome to þ eyes and syght. Also all euaporatyue

thyn=

thinges, as onions leekes, garlike mustarde, pease, and beanes, are very daungerous. Ye must kepe your feete cleane and forbeare the daye sleape. Beholde grene thynges, cleare water, precyous stones, and to kepe you from long holdyng downe youre face, socoureth the syghte verye moche, & is verye good for the eyes.

Lykewise vse meates of good & quicke digestion as to eate fenel often, and after meate take coriander confytes preparated, and drinke not after them.

But aboue al kepe away your handes for the rubbyng of them maketh them worse and worse.

¶ Remedie for diseases of the eares.

Take oyle of roses & a lytle vinegre, & putte it into the eare, then make a bagge of camomil & melilote, and laye it there vnto.

¶ For noyse and soundyng of the eares.

Take pillule cochie, or fetide, bycause

The regyment.

cause the founde proceedeth of ventofi
tie, or of phleyme, and before ye take
the fayde pylles, it is good to drynke
thre ounces of fenell water.ii. houres
before meate.iiii.or.v.dayes. After the
operation of the sayde pilles, ye muste
dyppe a tente in oyle of rue castor or of
salte, with the iuyce of leekes & often
in the mornynge fastynge to holde his
eare ouer the warme decoction of maiorym, rue, wormewood, camomil, and
mellilote.

¶ For peyne in the eares.

Gose grece wyth a lytle honye swageth the peynes of the eares.

¶ Also the chestwormes sodden in
oyle of rose vppon hote asshes in the
rinde of a pomegranate, and dropped
in the eares.

¶ Item oyle of almondes specially of
the bitter almons, hote.

¶ Item yf there be water in the eares
it shall be hadde oute wyth a litle gose
grese and the iuyce of onyons.

¶ Also earth wormes with gose grese
sodden

of lyfe.　　　Fol.xxi.

soden is good for payne in the eares. Item an adders hame soden in wyne and ye eare bathed in it, and a lytle therof put into the peyne is good to take a waye the gryefe, and it helpeth also to the eares that are rennyngt with stinkyng matter & corruption but in that case ye muste haue boyled in the wyne a lytle myrre.

⁋ Regyment.

The pacient muste eate and drynke lytle, and sweate in bathes, or whote houses, and sometymes to prouoke nesynge. He muste forbeare garlycke, onyons, leekes, pease, beanes, and nuttes, nor drynke wyne wythout water.

⁋ For deafnesse.

Sometyme there chaunceth deafnes by wynde, whyche is in the eare, the whyche causeth tynklynge in the head and then one muste put a litle aloes in hote water, or in whyte wyne, and distyll into the eare. Then put a lytle euphorbium in poudre into hys nose, to make hym to nese, & auoyde asmuche
humours

humours as ye can.

Some time deafenesse commeth of fleume, whych when it is olde is vncurable. But when it begynneth, it must be purged as hath ben said in the remedie of ỹ sounde of the eares. Thẽ take poudre of bay beries, and seth it ĩ oyle of lylies, and put it warme into your eare, and a lytle blacke wolle to stoppe the eare wyth, that no ayer entre.

Remedye for stynkyng of the nose.

Take cloues, gynger, and calamynte, of eche a lyke, & seethe thẽ in whyte wyne, and therewith washe thy nose. After put in poudre of piretrũ, to prouoke you to nese, & yf there be replecio̅ of fleume in the head, fyrst ye must purge it with pilles of cochie or of hiera picra. Also yf the cause of stinkyng come frõ the stomacke, fyrst helpe the stomacke, as shall be sayde hereafter in the remedies of the stomacke.

¶ Medicines for bleyng
of

of lyfe. Fol.xxii.
of the nose.

Take a dramme of boole armoniake wasshed, and myxte it in rosewater or plantayne water, and drynke it. Then bynde the extreme partes, as harde as ye may, and after make a tent of greke nettles, and put into his nose.

Moreouer, it is good for the pacyente to holde in his hande egremonie, with the rote and all, and drynke þ iuyce of knotgrasse, & without doubt þ blood shall staunche anon.

¶ For the same.

Set a boryng glasse vpon his lyuer, yf the blood come from the right syde, or on the splene, if he blede on the lefte syde & laye vnto the stones a good quā titie of towe or lynen dypped in vynegre, and for a woman laye it vpon her brestes.

¶ An other singuler medicine
for to staunche blood, and
it is a thynge experte of
al the good practitioners.

Take

The regyment

Take swynes dounge, euen as hote as ye can haue it from the swyne, and when ye haue clensed ye cōgeled bloud oute of the nose wrynge it thoroughe a cloute and let the iuyce perce into the side from whence the bloud commeth, and by the grace of God ye shall se it stanche anone

Moreouer it is good to bynd the fete and armes as harde as can be suffered, wyth a corde or a lace, the strōger they be bounde the better.

⸿ *Remedy for the tothe ache.*

PAyne of the tethe (as Galene sayeth) amōgest other paynes that are not mortall is ye most cruel and greuous of them all. It maye come dyuers wayes of a cold or hote cause. If it come of a hote cause his gomes are redde, and verye hote, wherfore it is verygood to holde i his mouthe water of camphore or to seeth a lytle camphore in vinegre, and holde it in his mouthe.

⸿ An other singuler remedye that
taketh

taketh awaye al kyndes of tothcache, specially yf it come of a hote cause.

Take henbane rootes, and seethe them in vynegre, and rosewater, & put the decoction in your mouthe.

Remedy for the tothache that commeth of colde causes.

For asmuche as in suche cases oftentymes there distilleth a boundaunce of water into ye mouth, purge it wt pillule cochie, and afterwardes kepe in youre mouth warme wyne, wherin hath ben sodden pellitore, myntes, and rewe.

¶ An other remedie for the same.

Take sage pellitorye, and seth them in vinegre, and kepe it in your mouthe as hote as ye maye suffer.

¶ An other for the same.

Take pellitorye, staue sacre, and the thre kyndes of pepper of eche one part macis, galigale, halfe parte of ye other make a poudre, and wyth a litle whyte wyne rubbe the teeth & then lay on ye foresayde pouder where the payne is.

An

The Regiment

¶ An other.

Take the myddle barke of an elder, salte, and pepper, of eche a like muche: and stampe them togither, and laye it to the sore teeth.

¶ An other remedye.

Take a lytle cotten, and dip it in oyle of spyke, thē put it on the sore tothe. If the tothe be hollowe, it is good to drawe it oute, for it wyll euerye daye wast what so euer ye do vnto it.

¶ To make the teeth whyte.

Take whyte marble, cuttle bone, whyte coral, sal gemme, baye salt, mastike, and pilles of a citron, of eche like moch, make them in very fine pouder, and rub the teeth therwith, euery mornynge. And afterwarde wasshe youre mouth with white wyne, wherin hath ben sodden a lytle cammomyl and dill.

¶ For the same.

Take vinegre of squilles and dippe a litle pyece of clothe in it, and rub the teeth and gummes withal. The sayde vinegre fastneth the gummes, comforteth

of lyfe.   Fol.xxiiii.

forteth the rotes of the teeth, & maketh a swete breath.

⁋ Another remedye to make
the teeth whyte.

Distylle a water in a lembik, of two partes of sallgēme, and ye thyrde part of alume, and rubbe the teeth wyth a lynnen cloute dypped in the same.

⁋ To take away stynkyng
of the mouthe.

Ye muste wasshe hys mouth wyth water and vynegre, & chewe mastike a good whyle, & then washe thy mouth wyth the decoctiō of anyse sedes, mintes, and cloues, sodden in wyne. If the stynkynge of the mouth commeth of a rottē tooth, the beste is to haue it drawen out.

⁋ Regymēt for tothe ache and,
stynkynge of the mouthe.

Ye muste wasshe your mouth, before and after meat with warme water for to clense the mouthe, and to purge the humours from the gommes which desfende out of the head. It is good euery
mornyng

mornyng fastig, to washe your mouth and to rubbe þ teeth with a sage lefe, pilles of citron, or wyth pouder made of cloues & nutmygges. Ye muste forbere lettuce, rawe frute, al tarte metes and the chewyng of hard thynges. Also all meates of euell digestion, and vomytynge.

⸿ The thyrde chapter treateth of remedyes for diseases of the breaste.

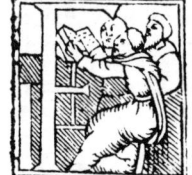

Fyrst for hoareenes of the voice, that maketh a man to speke lowe, & wyth great peine ye must auoyde al egre salte, & sharpe thiges, & sleping by daye, to moch watchig great colde muche speakyng, & to loude cryeng. Al swete thinges are very good as apples sodden with suger great rausins, fygges, almonde mylke, hulled barlye, pignolate, penedies, whyte pylles, sugre candye, and

of lyfe.   fol.xxv

and the iuyce of licorice.

¶ Remedye for a hoarce voyce.

Take the broth of redde colewortes, and myngle wyth it .vii. or .viii. penydyes, & an ounce of syrupe of mayden heare, and gyue vnto the pacient, when he goeth to bedde.

¶ An other medicine.

Take diapris simple, & eate a lozenge of the same at morne & also at nyght.

¶ Another remedy for hoarcenes of a long contynuaunce.

Take great raysons, fygges, suger cinamome, and cloues, of euerye one a litle. Seeth them in good wyne, of the which ye shal gyue to drynke mornyng & euenyng .ii. ounces at a time, except he hath a feuer.

¶ For the same.

It is good to take mornyng and euenyng, a sponefull of the syrupe of iuiubes mixte wyth a roote of liquyrice, in maner of aloe. If wyth the sayd hoarcenes, there descende aboundaunce of water to the mouth, it is good to make an

Di.   electuarye,

electuarye, of halfe diapris, and halfe diadragantum, & to vse it first & last, after perfuminge wt stoupes of flaxe, fumed wyth frankinsence, mastik, candrake, and storax calamite, laide vpon the head warme

Remedye for the cough.

Take ysope, great raysins, and figges, of eche a lytle handefull, licorice one ounce, boile them in water till the third parte be wastid, then giue it him for to drynke twyse a daye, i the mornyng two houres before meate, and at nyghte one houre before supper, and immedialye after, it is good to eate a lozenge of diairis, or diapenidion. If ye wyll haue it stronger put to them, i the decoction a little coole woortes, anyse, and fenell, wyth the sedes of nettelies, of eche .ii. drammes.

¶ An other remedie.

Take suger candye, whyte pylles of siris, & diadragagant, of euery one .i. ounce, licorice ii. drammes, make a pouder, and let hym eate therof a sponful, mornynge

of lyfe.　　Fo.xxvi

morninge and euenyng, and drynke after it three ounces of water of Isope, or of scabiouse, with sugre or without suger.

In stede of those waters, ye maye take the brothe of redde colewoortes wythout salte.

　　An other remedye.
Take sirupe of liquirice, and of ysope and drynke it euen and morne, wyth a ptisane or one of ý same sirupes, with a sponeful of ptisane is good.

¶ In other.
Take pouder of diapnis simple, and liquirice of eche a dramme weyghte, & with .iiii. ounces of suger make an electuarye, to be eaten fyrste and last, and after meate.

¶ In other
It is good to take loesanum, with a stycke of liquirice, at the coughynge, and after meate. And there is an other loc called loc de pino, as good at all tymes as the other is. And it is good to annoint the breast mornynge and eue-

　　D ii.　　　　nynge,

The regyment

nynge, wyth oyle of lillies, swete almons, and maye butter wythout salte.

Here is to be noted, that commonlye ye coughe procedeth of colde humours that greueth the longes, and for that cause all thynges the whyche be hote, swete, and do prouoke spittel, are very good and holsome for the same, as be the thynges afore rehersed.

And sometyme it procedeth of heate, & then it is knowen by the great alteration or feuer & then ye muste forbydde ye pacient drynkynge of all wynes, & to vse the thynges ye hereafter foloweth.

¶ Remedye agaynst the cough commyng of a hote cause.

Take sirupe of vyolettes, and of iuiubes, and drynke therof mornyng & euenyng, with a lytle ptisane sodden,
¶ For the same.

It is good to take fyrste and laste, a lozenge of diadragagant, & afterwarde to drinke a dreught of good ptisane,
¶ A good receypte agaynst the coughe.

D.iii,   Take

of lyfe.　　fol. xxvi

Take the rote of Enula campana, horehounde, holihock, of eche a lyke moche, seeth them altogyther, in whyte wyne wyth a dosen of fatte fygges, and a lytle liquirice, drynke of it a draught, euerye daye twyse,

C Regiment or dyet for them
　　that haue the cough.

Ye must abstayne from vynegre, vertuce all salte meates, frutes, and rawe herbes, fysshe, lymons, grosse meates, and to muche repletion. Also ye maye drinke no wyne betwene meales, and beware of daye slepe, and specially after meate.

The wynde, the colde, and muche talkynge, are verye vnnaturall for the cough, and so is all laboure aswell of the bodye as of the mynde, and sometyme it is good to holde your wynde a lytle, and let it go agayne.

　　C Remedyes agaynst
　　　Shortnes of the
　　　　wynde.
　　　　　　　Shortnes

The Regyment

Shortnes of the wind procedeth oftentymes of fleume, that is tough and clammishe, hangynge vpon ẏ longes or stoppinge ẏ condits of ẏ same, beinge in the holowenes of the brest, or of catarrous humours ẏ droppeth downe into the longes, and thereby cōmeth straitnesse in drawing of the breth, whych is called of phisitions dispnoea or asthma, & whan ẏ pacient can not bend his necke down for dredc of suffocation it is called orthopnoea. For euerye one of these diseases there be very holsome medicines declared here afore.

☙ The receypte for Asthma.

Take an ounce of great raisins picked from the kernelles, two figges the meat of a date, dry isope, maydenhere, licorice, and the longes of a foxe washed in wyne, water of scabiouse, of euery one a dramme, penidies, 2. ounces with sirupe of licorice let al be scorporated, & make aloe, to eat a good while after meate, wyth a sticke of lycorice.

Another

of lyfe.　　fol.xxviii

¶ In other receypte.

Take horehounde, maydenhere, and ysope, of euery one a handful, liquirice dates fygges, seed of smalache, and of fenell of euery one half an ounce, boyle them in a pinte of water and an halfe tyll the thyrde parte be consumed. After gyue hym the sayde decoction, to drinke a good draught euery mornyng two houres afore meat And before it, or incontinentlye after it, it is good to take asmoche as a chesnut of conserue of colewortes, or a lozenge of dyaysopi or diairis Salomonis. Also loc de pulmone vulpis, is excedynge good for ye sayde disease.

¶ An ointment for shortnes of breath
Take, ti ounces of oyle of swete almōdes, one of maye butter vnsalted, a lytle saffron, and of newe waxe, & make an oyntmente, wherewith ye shall annoynte the brest morne and euen.

¶ Regiment.
Consideryng ye sayde disease commeth of to great aboūdaunce of fleume
in the

in the longes, it is good to obserue the thinges that are shewed in the remedyes of the cough. And to dwell in a drye place farre from water pooles, or marishes, and to slepe in a moyste chābre, in the whiche ye muste haue a fyre of wood without smoke. The bread must be lyght and pleasaunt, for soure bread browne bread, and crustes, are to be auoyded. Also ye maye eate no peace, beanes, nuttes, chesnuttes, nor any thyng that stoppeth or engendreth wynde.
Fysshe rosted vpon the grydyron maye well be suffred for they be not so euyl. Hulled barly, ryse, broth of colewoortes, and broth of an olde cocke with Isope & saffron, are speciall good meate for the longes, and so are fatte fygges raysins of alican, dates, graynes of ye pyne, pignolate, and swete almondes. Great mouynges and chafynges, and sodayne laboure is verye euyll, yet moderat exercyse afore meate is good & profytable.
Reunynge, angre, and suche other passions

of lyfe. fol.xxix.

sions that enflame the hert, are in this case vtterly to be auoyded

⁋Remedyes for the pthisycke.

Phisis is an vlceration of the longes, by the which el the body falleth into consumption, in suche wyse that it wasteth al saue the skyn. Ye maye knowe hym that hath a pthisicke, for from day to day he waxeth euer leaner and dryer, and hys hear falleth, and hath euer a cough, and spitteth so mtyme mater and bloody strynges wythall. And yf ẏ whyche he spytteth be put ito a basyn of water it falleth to ẏ bottome, for it is so heauye.

Galene speakyng of this dysease, sayeth it is vncurable. But when he was i Rome, he gaue counsayle to thē that had the pthysickes, to dwel in the mountaynes and hye places, far from waters, & watry groūdes, and so theyr lyfe shulde be prolonged but at the last they dyed of the same disease. Neuerthelesse, it is good to release the payne, and to helpe them as much as it is possible.

The regyment

sible. And the thynge that is moste holsome for the same, is to drynke euerye mornyng a draught of asses milke, iiii. houres afore meate, in the place wherof one maye take the milke of a goote, newlye milked, and mixe them euerye tyme with a sponeful of poudre, made of sugre of roses. And it is good euery tyme to vse cōserue of roses, pignolat diadragagantū, and annoynt the brest before and behynd, wyth oyle of swete almondes, maye butter, and salte.

¶ An other remedy proued by a religious man.

¶ Take two ounces of pimpernell in poudre, and therof make an electuarye wt sugre, & vse it euery mornyng. ii. drāmes with pimpernel water. iii. oūces. Water of snaples distilled, is proued good to them that be pthisyke, euerye mornynge in drinke, & for al them that are drye & leane.   ¶ An other.

¶ Take the. iiii. colde seedes, seede of quinces, of eche. iii. drāmes and a halfe whyte poppe seed. v. drāmes, the iuce

of

of lyfe.　　fol.xxxi

of liquirise, ysope, amidum, gūme ara=
bike, and dragant, of eche a dramme
and an halfe, penidies, the weyghte of
them all, make a poudre, and vse euery
morninge .ii. drammes, and after take
two sponefulles of syrupe of iuiubes
or i stede of it drinke the ptisan of wa=
ter of vngula caballina, otherwyse cal
led horsehofe. The poudre whereof is
good for the pthisike, wherewyth Ha
ly sayth, that he heled a mōke, of the
same sycknesse.

¶ Regiment for pthisyke
Ye ought to do as hath ben sayde in
regimente of Asthma, and to abstayne
from all spices, saue saffron. Ye muste
lykwyse abstayne from all sowre thin
ges, sharpe thynges, & tarte nor be not
hungry, nor drye: but cherysh you well
with meates of easie digestion, & good
norischmente, suche as is coleps of ca=
pons, hulled barlye, almon mylke, eg=
ges yolkes, veale, kydde, lambe, shepes
fete, and small birdes liuing in wodes
and busshes, creauises & fysshe of swete
　　　　　　　　runnyng

The regymment
runnyng water, hauyng scales. Snaylles in the shelles sodde wyth fenell and ysope, is very good. Ye must lyue merily, & playe at some pastyme for pleasure, wythout labouring. He oughte to abstayne from laxatiue medicines, bycause that it is sayde. Cum fluor crecedit, mors intrat, vita recedit, whiche is contrarye to asthma, for therein it is good euer to be lose bellyed.

⁋ For the pleuresye.

Hereafter shalbe spoken of medicynes for diseases of the ribbes. And for playner knowlege of the same, ye shall vnderstande that sometime in the skinnes that couer the rybbes, there gathereth togyther bloud and cholerycke humours, which engendre apostemes called pleuresie, & it maye be knowen by iiii. maner of sygnes. Fyrst the paciente hath a great burnyng feuer. Secondly the ribbes are so sore within, as if they were prycked continually wt nedylles. Thyrdly, the pacient hath a shorte breathe. The .iiii. sygne is a strōg cough, where

of lyfe. fol.xxvii

wherewyth the sycke is vexed, and by these sygnes maye ye surelye knowe a ryght pleuresie, that is the skyn vnder the rybbes wythin the bodye.

But there is an other kynde of pleuresie wythout vpon the rybbes apostemed, but in that is nothyng so greatte daunger nor the fyeuer is not so strōg as is the other aforerehearsed.

¶ Remedye.

The paciente oughte to be let bloud on the liuer veyne, in the cōtrary arme from ẏ syde that is diseased. After the begynnynge of the sore, tyll the thyrde daye, and after that yf the paciente be not feble, let hym bloud agayne vpō ẏ same syde, that the sore is. Moreouer, the pacient ought to laye vpō the sore syde, euery daye an earthen bottel full of warme water, and to annoynte his rybbes with oyle of camompl warme. And he ought to take a glyster of chyckyns brothe, mylke, cassia, oyle of vyolettes, and hony of roses, yf his bellye be harde. And in stede of that glister, it
is good

The Regiment

is good to take ã osice of cassia, i. houre before dinner, in a lozenge, oz destempered wyth a ptisane, oz els wyth water of scabiouse.

¶ An other remedy.

Take of bromefloures, of scabiouse and the great thistle called cardo benedictus, of euery one a like portiõ, medle them togyther, and let him euerye morninge and euening, receyue a good draught, and annoint the ribbes with oile of bromflours, and it shalbe good

¶ An other singuler remedy.

Take. iii. ounces of water of oure ladye thystle, one sponefull of whyte wyne, and syxe inner whytes of egges well brayed, myngle all togither, and laye them playsterwyse vppon the ribbes, as hote as ye maye suffre.

¶ An other experte remedye.

Take. ii. good handfulles of horsdong two racis of gynger in pouder, & then wrappewell the donge & the ginger together in a clene linen cloth, then putte them of lyfe. fol.xxv

them in a newe potte to boyle wyth.ii. pintes of whyte wyne, vntyl ye thyrd parte be consumed, & drinke a draught of the sayde drynke euery morninge, & after ye haue dronke the sayd wine couer ye aswel as is possible & sweate.

℟ Regyment for the pleuresy.

The patient ought not to drink wine nor eate flesche, but muste be cōtent to drinke ptisane, barli water and weake drynke, & to eate barly hulled, & milke of almons clarefied, rosted apples and great raisins as longe as ye feuer doth last. And for to helpe hym to spyt, it is good to vse often white pilles, diadragagantū, suger candye, and other thinges sayde in the remedye of the cough.

℟ For diseases in the ribbes whiche is not pleuresie.

There chaunceth often tymes a disease in the rybbes, whyche they call a bunche, whych commeth of ventositie wherfore it is good to apply therto hote thinges, as a toste of bread very hot & a lytle bagge of otes, & baye salt fryed

The Regiment

ed togyther, or of hony whyche is better. Also it shall be good to put therto a sponefull of hote asshes and herbes, of horehounde, rue, wormewode, margerym, ysope, bayes, and camomylle.

⁋ Another remedy for the same

Take the rotes of colewort & hoppes of eche an ounce, vervayne, mugworte, sage, myntes wormewood, tansaye, and motherworte, of eche a handefull, put all in a commen stylle and dystylle them.

Kepe that water to drynke, euerye mornynge. ii. or. iii. ounces, whyle the peyne doth laste.

⁋ Another remedye.

Take the sayde herbes and rootes, & beate them with whyte wyne, & streine them thorow a linnent clothe, and gyue vnto the patient a smalle draught. ii. or iii. houres afore meate.

⁋ The fourth Chapiter of the weakenes of the harte.

Weakenes

of lyfe. Fo. xxxiiii.

Weakenesse or feblenes of hert is caused when the bodye fayleth his vertue vital, without anye euident cause or whē the bodye is cōsumed, and waxeth out of colour, & that the operations vitall are weake, wythout sensible hurtynge of any other mēbre, but the hart. And it may chaunce of an aposteme, for the whiche there is no maner remedy, for al apostematiō of the hart is mortal.

And debilitie of the harte may come of heate accidentall, whiche one maye know when there is great heate in the breast, and vehement thirst, and is quēched better in drawing colde ayre, then in drynkyng colde water.

¶ Remedye.

Gyue him ẏ hath a feble hert, & redy to faint, either for feuer or for extreme heate, the weyght of a frenche crowne of trosciske of cāphore, with wyne of pomegranades, & laye vpon hys breast towarde the lefte syde, a cenda or lynnen

E.i.

The Regiment

nen dipped in water of roses & vinegre
¶ lectuarye.

In stede of these troseishes, ye maye vse a lectuary called diamargaritō frigidū, euerye mornyng a lozenge. And it is good to gyue him for þ same feblenes conserue roses, violettes, & water lillies, myngled togyther, and after to drynke water of sorell, & to smel roses, water lilies, rose water, and vinegre.

Otherwhyles and most often, debilitie of harte chaunceth of a colde and drye cause, and is wythout feuer, with great feare and heuynesse, the remedye whereof is thys.

Remedye.

Take of an electuarye called diamuscus, or of another called electuarium pliris, and vse euery mornyng a lozenge, and drynke after it a lytle good wyne, or buglosse water: & annoynte the breaste wyth ople of spykenarde. Moreouer vse ones i a weke fyue houres before meate: the weight of halfe a crowne of good triacle or mithridatū
so it

of lyfe.　　fol.xxxiiii.

so it be wel tempered in a lytle whyte wyne, wyth a few maces.

⁋For the same.

Ye muste gyue the pacient often in the houre of hys feblenesse, cloues, cynamome, nutmygges, setuale, of the roote of colewortes, yf he hathe not ye phthisycke, in whyche case he must absteyne from the said thinges. And it is conueniente to gyue hym in that case, good fleshe, & potage without spices & take euery mornig, a great draught of asses or goates milke, & suger rosate.

⁋For beatyng of the harte.

It is called of the physicians cardiaca passio, or otherwyse tremor cordis, that is tremblyng of hart, & sometime it chaunceth wyth a feuer, & sometyme wythout.

⁋Remedye whan it commeth wyth a feuer.

Ye muste be let bloode of the lyuer vayne and drynke euery mornynge syrupe of pomgranades, & lymmons, the iuce of sorelle, or of one of them, wyth

E.ii.　　　water

The regyment

water of roses, purcelane, succorye, & sorelle. Moreouer the paciēt ought to smell thynges co de and swete, as dryed roses, water lilies, violettes & vinegre of roses.

Also it is good to take an infusiō or lare of reubarbe, ordeined of som good phisition, after the whyche it shall be good, to applye vpon the lefte pappe, a lynnen cloth dypped in plataine water, roses, sorell, and a lytle vinegre.

¶ For tremblyng of the hart without a feuer, a remedye.

The pacient must take .ii. drammes of the electuarye of diamargariton calidum, and the thyrde part of electuarium de gemmis, then drynke .ii. or .iii. ounces of water of buglosse & bawme mixt together.

¶ An other remedye.

Take mastyke, lignum aloes, cloues, cynamome, nutmygges, and cubebes of eche a scruple, pylles of citrons halfe a dramme, doronici romani, and yles, of eche .xv. graynes, basile seede,

ten

of lyfe.　　Fol.xxxv.

ten graynes, ambre grece, and muske, of eche .ii. graynes, with conserued bugloſſe, or colewortes and sucket of cytrons, of eche halfe an ounce, make an electuarye wyth .iiii. ounces of suger diſſolued in whyte wyne, and bugloſſe water, and vſe of the same euery mornynge .ii. drammes, and drynke a lytle good wyne after it

¶ Another remedye.
Take water of bugloſſe, bawme, and borage, of all thre togyther a pounde, of white wyne halfe a pounde, pouder of cinamome, cloues and nutmygges, of eche two drammes, myngle them al wel togyther, and then heate it a litle, and dyppe a lynnen cloth in it, or els a scarlette, & laye it to the left pappe.

¶ Another remedye.
Ye muſte make a bagge of sendalle, of the sayde swete spyces, or other cordyal pouders and laye it hote vpō the lefte pappe.

An other remedye.
Take pomaunders made of laydanum,

E.iii.

The Regyment

num, lignum aloes, and citron pylles, maces, cloues, boragz floures, storax calamite, ambre of grece, and a lytle waxe, and let the pacient beare that & smell it often.

¶ An other medicyne.

The mawe of an olde cocke dryed and made in pouder is excedinge good to drynke in red wyne or swete wyne wyth a lytle safron.

¶ For the same.

It is good to drynke euerye mornynge thre ouces of water of buglosse, wherein hath bene sodden cloues. And it is good to drynke in a mornynge .iii. ouces of iulep, made of halfe a pound of bawme water, and .iii. ounces of suger. The confection of dialacincthi, is singuler and excellent for tremblynge of the harte, but it is for noble men not for poore folke.

¶ For swownyng.

Swowning is a takynge away of the felynge and mouyng of the body, by weaknes of the hart, thorough of lyfe. Fol.xxxvi

tough to moch auoydans of the spirites. ¶Remedye.

In fwomen for fownynge, sodenly ye ought to cast into hys face colde water myngled with rosewater or vinegre. And yf ye stoppe hys mouth, and nose and bowe hys face vnto hys knees so lõge as ye stoppe your winde your selfe ye shall forthwyth recouer hym. But yf the sayde swownynge come of the mother, ye muste laye to the nose al stynkynge thynges, and abhominable sauours, as partriches fethers brente, castor, and assafetida, or the snuffes of candelles. Moreouer ye ought to gyue the pacient a litle good wyne, which is the chefe thynge that quycklyest restoreth hym, as sayth Auerrois in hys seuenth colliget. Afterwarde rubbe his armes and legges, and bynde them harde then prouoke hym to nese, puttynge a lytle pouder of longe pepper, euphorbium, or castor, into hys nose. And yf by the sayde medicines the pacient doth not

E.iiii. amende,

amende, this disease is uncurable.

And here ye may note, that yf swowning come by great resolution of spirites, as after great euacuation, other by swette, flure of bloud, or laxe, ye ought not to cast cold water on his face, nor to bynd his mēbres, for ħ shuld do him hurt, but kepe hym in a place wythout mouynge, & gyue hym to drynk a lytle good wyne, & nourishe him with good light meates, as pullettes, chickyns, capons, partriches, veale, muttō, & kyd. Whereof ye may make him good porrege, colepses, or restoratyues, distilled or otherwise as ye shal thike coueniēt.

¶ The .v. Chapter, of remedyes for diseases of the stomake.

The cheste of ħ bodye doth receyue ħ meate necessarye for al the mēbres in the stomake whiche is situate i the myddes of the bodye for to digest the same meate into al the mēbres, to the which chaūceth debilitie, or hyndrans of appetite, some times by errour of ħ eater in qua

of lyfe. Fo.xxxviii.

in qualitie or quātitie, & somtymes by reason of the reume that descendeth from the head lyke a reume.

¶ Remedye

Kepe abstinence, and eate soberlye lyght meates, and drynke good wyne, and but litle. Purge the stomake, in takynge pylles of symple hiera before meate. iii. or foure of the sayd pilles at foure of the clocke in the mornyn~. If the repletion be greate, sleppynge in the nyght he muste laye hys hande on hys stomake, or els laye a lytle pyllowe of fethers on it, or a bagge of wormwood & margerym. Sometymes there chaunceth suche debilitie, not for reume, or meate or drike, but by viscouse and slymy fleume, i the mouth of the stomake which causeth to engedre aboūdaūce of ventosítie, and maketh the meate to swymme wyth lytle thyrst. And sometymes with sour belchinges: and inflations, suche debilitie maye not perfitely be cured, but for a tyme mēded, with the remedyes that folowe.

Reme

The Regiment

⁋ Remedyes for weakenesse of the stomake

Fyrst ye must take pillule stomatice ii. or iii. houres afore meat more or lesse accordynge to ye quantitie of the fulnesse of the stomake, & after giue hi euery mornyng .ii houres afore meate, and one houre after supper, at euery tyme a lozenge of a Iectuary called diagalāga, or an other called diaciminō, whyche Iectuaryes do consume ventosities, & wyth theyr comfortable heate, dryue awaye the colde and the wyndye complexion of the stomacke.

⁋ For the same.

Grene gynger is verye good taken as is sayd afore of electuaryes. And it is holsome to eate afore your meate, anyse seedes & fenell, whē ye begyn to eate, take a tost dipped in soddē wine, or good malucsey wythout drynkynge of the same wyne, except it be a very little after meate.

⁋ Another.

Take mastyke and lapdanū, of euery

of lyfe.   Fol.xxix

rye one an ounce, myntes, and wormewood poudred, of eche a dramme, turbentyne as moche as shall nede to encorporate them togither, make a playster and sprede it vpon lether, and laye it to the stomake. In stede of the sayde plaister, it is good to annoynte the stomake with oyle of spikenarde, and mastyke, or to laye on it hoote breade steped in good wyne, on the which bread strowe pouder of cloues & nutmygges.

Sometymes suche debilitie of stomake cōmeth of hote causes, & thē it is knowen by the litle appetite to meate, and great thryste, and head ache before meate, and after it, cōmeth stynkynge belchyng, wherof sometyme soloweth vomytyng, and is holpe on this wise.

⸿ Remedye.

If in suche debilitie if there be great quantitie of spyttle, and muche desyre to vomyte, it is good to take x. drammes of hiera piera, wyth the decoction of cycers, or with two or thre ouces of water of wormewood, and after your meate

The regiment

meate vse coriander seed prepared, and beware ye drynke not thereafter, nor slepe in the day tyme.

¶ To the same.

Mirabolanes condite are very good for the same purpose, to begyuen ones in the weke, at four of the clocke i the mornig, halfe an ounce or a hole ouce euery tyme, and take awaye the stone that is within. If in the sayd debilitie of stomake of hoote cause, there be not aboūdaunce of spyttle, but dryness of mouth, with thyrst & vomytyng, stynkyng & fumyshe, it is good to take euery mornynge syrupe of sorel, syrupe of roses, or sirupe of quices, with endiue and succorye water, or water sodden and cooled againe, and thē drinke hiera picra, as afore is said, or take a purgation as is declared in the payne of the head, cōmynge of cholere. It is to be noted, that for suche debilitie of the stomake, ye may not weare any cerote playster, nor bagge, wherin is hote medicines lest ye shulde augmēt the cause
but

of lyfe. Fol. xi.

but it is conuenient to annoynt the
stomake wyth colde oyles, as be oyles
of roses, and quinces, and yf ye wyll
haue a playster, make it of redde roses
and saunders.

⁋ For abhorryng of meate.

Ometyme there chaunceth in
the stomake, a disease called
fastidium, or abhorynge of
meate whereby the person a-
gaynst his wil, taketh in hate and ab-
hominacion all maner of meates, that
is offered vnto hi, lykewyse as a hole
man taketh pleasure and delyte in his
meate. The cause of this disease, is re-
plecio of cholericke humours, or phleg-
matike, grosse and viscouse, w[hi]ch are
in the stomake, & the patiēt hath great
thyrste, a drye tonge, the mouth bytter,
& sometime doth vomyt yelowe cholere.

⁋ Remedye.

Ye muste purge the cholere as hath
bene sayde afore, and yf the veynes be
greate and ful of bloud, ye ought to let
him bloud on the right arme, & on that
veyne

veyne whiche appeareth moost, and to quycken ye appetite it is good to gyue him to eate or drinke, such as the pacient demaūdeth, although it be not alwayes of the best. And also it is good to gyue him ye iuce of pomegranades.

For belchynge.

Belchyng is a ventositie inflatiue, expulsed out of the stomake to the mouth, and commeth by feblenes, and litle heat of the stomake, which engendreth wynde, wherfore it signifieth a colde complexion, whiche is cause of suche ventositie after meate. And for this disease ye shall do as foloweth.

Remedye for wyndynesse of the stomake.

Abstayne from all frutes, and rawe herbes, pease, beanes, garlike, onyons, leekes, chesnuttes, course meates, great repast, and slepe on the daye. Ye ought to take fastynge, cōfytes made of aneys, fenell, cummyne, and carreway seedes, or els pouder of the sayde thynges mixte wyth suger. Also it is
good

good to take ĩ a mozninge two houres before meate, a lozenge of aromaticum rosatũ, ⁊ yf ye haue an akyng stomake and colde, it is good to take euery moznyng a lozẽge of dianisi, oz diaciminũ oz some other cõfoztable lozenge, ⁊ to dzike after it a sponeful of good wine

⁋ An other remedye.
Ye may take a lytle galingale, with a litle wine, oz pouder of cumyne with some good wyne.

⁋ An other remedye.
Dzynke euery moznyng fastyng, two ounces of wyne wherin hath bene sodden baye beries, anyse, ⁊ carreway seedes, of eche a lytle. And yf ye put to it a litle pure frankensence, it wolde be the better. And wythout, it is good to laye a bagge full of camomyll floures, rue, woznewoode, ⁊ maiozym made in pouder, oz foz to annoynte the stomake with oyle of woznewoode, rue, syknard, oz bayes.

Somtymes suche belchyng and vẽtositie cõmeth befoze meate, and it is
caused

The regiment.

caused of fleume viscouse, or watrisshe, that is in the stomake.

¶ Remedye.

Ye must purge the fleume with pilluse cochie, or electuarium of diacartami, as hath ben sayd in the remedye of peine of the heed caused of fleume. And ere ye gyue the purgatiō, ye ought. iii. or. iiii. mornynges two houres afore meate, to take two lytle sponefulles of syrupe of wormewood, or of myntes.

After the whyche purgation, it is good to annoynt þ stomake wh oyle of mastike, nardine, wormewood or lilies and for to weare vpō the stomake a cerote being made lyke a playster, which ye maye bye at the Apotecaris, called cerotum Galeni, or a bagge made of maiorim, and camompl floures, & take euery mornyng a lozenge of the electuary abouenamed, or of diagalanga.

Item ye shal note, that yf the person can not take a purgatiō, to auoyde suffieyently the fulnesse of the stomake, which hyndreth the digestion of meate

he must

of lyfe.   Fol.xlii

he muſt take a glyſter, and afterward pilles of elephangine, or of hiera ſimplicis, before dynner or ſupper. Moreouer, yf before dynner ye fele an heuyneſſe in the ſtomake, ye oughte to take one of the ſayde pylles: halfe an houre before meate.

⁋For the hycket.

Hycket or yeaſkyng, is an euyll mouyng of the vertue expulſiue of the ſtomake prouoked by the vertue ſenſible, to expulſe that that doeth anoye. The ſayd hicket doth ſomtimes happen by reaſon of emptyneſſe, by debilitie of ye ſtomake after long ſykneſſe, or by flux of blud or lax, or by ſome other ſtrãge euacuation, which is very perylous & oftẽtimes mortal. Therfore it is good to gyue reſtoratiues to the patient, & to giue him ſofte egges, almon mylke, hulled barly, cullepes of capons, or other thynges of good noryſhment, and of eaſye digeſtion.

Alſo ye ought to ſtoppe the lare, & to make ye patient to ſlepe longe, and an
            F   noynte

noynte the stomake with oyle of swete almons. Sometimes hicket procedeth of repletiō of matter humorous, or of drīke and meate which engēdre grosse ventositie, & not very easy to cōsume. Yf þ stomake be ouer charged w̄ meates kepe a long abstinēce til digestiō be done, or els vomit and annoint thy stomake with oyle of dyll, mastik, wormewood & castor. If humours cōtened in the stomake be cause of the said hicket take ā ounce of hierapicra w̄ water of wormwood or els pilles āte cibū. iii or 4. houres before meat, & euerie morning folowing þ operatiō of þ said hierapicra, take a lozēge of dianisi or diaciminum, or els a fewe anys seedes & carawayes

C Regyment for all maner hyckette.

It is good to kepe long and often his breath, to neese, to trauayle moche, to endure greate thyrst, and also to sleape long: And it is good to caste colde water in the face of him that hath the hicket:c, and to threaten him, and so put hym of lyfe.　　　fol. xliii.

hym in feare, & to angre hym, or els to prouoke him to heuynes, for by these thynges the naturall heate is reuoked and fortifyed within, and causeth the hycket to cease.

For vomiting.

Vomtyng commeth somtymes wt out great vyolence, & therby one getteth health, wherfore ye nede not gyue him any remedie, for it is a good actiō of the naturall vertue of the stomake. Sometyme vomtynge commeth by a great violent mouyng of the vertue expulsyue of the stomacke, for the euyll thynges conteyned in the same.

Remedye.

One maye well helpe a man to vomyte, gyuing hym warme water with a lytle oyle to drynke, or els to put the fynger in his mouth very lowe, or a fether wette in oile, the better to vomite and mundifye the stomake, yf so be the persone haue a wyde throte, and that vomiting do not hurte hym moche, as be they that haue but smal and strayte

F.ii.　　　　　　　throtes

The regyment

throtes, and longe neckes and leane, ⁊ he that hath an euyl syght, for al these it is euyll to vomyte,

Sometymes vometyng commeth by weakenesse of þ stomacke, caused of a hote and euil complexion, ye shal heale it after this maner.

℣ Remedye.

Take sirupe of roses, quynces, myrtylles, wyth water sodden, and colde agayne, or elles water of purcelane for to refresshe and quenche the thyrst þ chaunceth commonlye in suche a case, And it is good to annoynt þ stomake before dynner ⁊ supper, wyth an oyntment made of oyle of roses, and quinces, wyth iuyce of myntes, and a lytle waxe, or els to make a playstre of mintes, roses, wormewood, ⁊ oile of roses and laye it to the stomake.

℣ An other.

Take frakensence, mastike, of eche halfe an ounce made ī pouder, and mē gle them togyther, with the whyte of an egge, and a lytle barlye floure, then
spred

of lyfe. fol. xliii

spyede it on a lytle towe, and laye it to the mouth of the stomake. At the latter ende of diner, it is good to take a mor sell of marmalade wythout drynke.

Somtyme vometinge procedeth of euyll & colde complexion of the stomake
⁋ Remedye.
Anoynt the stomake with oyle of spik narde and mastike, orels make on oint ment of the sayde oyles, wyth a lytle mastyke, corall, and waxe, and anoynt the stomake mornyng and euenynge.

⁋ An other medicine.
Make a bagge of wormewood, ma iorym, and drye myntes, of eche a litle handfull, cloues, galingale, & nutmyg ges, of eche halfe a dramme, the sayde thynges poudred, and put betwyxt ii. linen clothes with cotten enterbasted and applied vpon the stomacke, are of wonderfull operation. In sted of this ye maye take the sayd herbes dried on an hote tilestone, and put them in two lynnen cloutes vpon the stomake.

⁋ An other maner.

F.iiii.   ye

The Regyment.

Ye maye take a toste of bꝛeed & stepe it in the iuce of myntes, and cast vpō it pouder of mastyke, then lape it vpō the stomacke, and from thꝛe houres to thꝛe houres let it be renewed.

⁋ Otherwyse.

Take two handfulles of mintes, and a handfull of roses sodde in wyne, thā take two ounces of tosted bꝛeed, and moyste it in wyne, and incoꝛpoꝛate it with pouder of mastike, and the sayde roses & myntes, and make a playster, whereof one parte must be layed to ye stomake when the patient wolde eate anye meate. The sayde playster is also good in all hote causes, yf foꝛ the saide wyne, ye seeth the myntes and roses, and stepe the toste in vinegre.

⁋ To comfoꝛt the stomake after vomytynge.

It is good to gyue vnto the pacient euerye moꝛnyng an ounce of sirupe of woꝛmewood, oꝛ myntes, in steade of which it is cōuenient to take a loꝛēge of aromaticū rosatum, oꝛ diagalāga

fo.

of lyfe.　　Fol. xlb

¶ For the same.

Take euenynge and moꝛnyng .iii. houres before meate, ii. cloues in pouder, wyth a sponefull of the iuce of mintes oꝛ halfe a sponefull of rue, dꝛyed wyth a lytle wyne.

Also it is good to take poudꝛe of clones and lignum aloes the weyght of a crowne, wyth wyne, ii. houres before meate.

¶ A glystre for the same.

And here ye muste note, that in all vomptyng, yf the patient be harde bellyed, it is good to take a lenitiue glistre made of the decoction of marche mallowes, mallowes, violettes, and barly with oyle of violettes, honie of roses, and a litle cassia. And yf the vompting come of coldnes of ẏ stomake, oꝛ of cold water cōteyned ī it, adde vnto the said glyster, woꝛmwood, ysope, rue, and cammomylle in the sethynge. And for oyle of violettes, take oyle of camomil oꝛ of lylyes, and gyue the patient a pil of mastyke befoꝛe meate. And ye shall

F. iiii.　　vnder

The regyment

vnderstande, that myntes brayed, and myngled wyth oyle of roses, and applyed vpon the stomake, is verie good for all vomiting.

¶ For peyne of the stomake.

Ache or peyne of the stomake commeth somtimes of wynde, and it is called dolour extensyue, the which is holpen with applyig therto a sponge wet in wyne, wherei hath ben soddē wormwood, rue and camomyll.

Also ye may helpe it as hath ben sayd in the remedy of hycket or yeaskynge, and as shalbe sayd hereafter in the remedy for all peynes of the stomake.

Sometymes the sayde payne commeth of repletiō of humours, and it is called dolor aggrauatiuus. Whyche ought to be cured by purgation, in gyuing of cassia newly drawen out, hiera picra, or pylles stomaticas, or of hiera simple, takyng some syrupe before the purgation, as is shewed in the remedy of debilitie of stomake.

Sometymes payne of the stomake cōmeth

of lyfe. fol.xlvi.

meth of cholere, oɿ salte fleume verye sharpe, and ẏ patient hath bytter tast oɿ salt with great thirst, and he fealeth heate and moɿdiratiõ. Wherfoɿe it is good to dɿynke sirupe of roses, oɿ occi saccarũ simple w̃ soddẽ water & coled.

In stede wherof ye may take endiue water, succoɿye and purcelane, wyth one parte of woɿmewood water, and then take an euacuatyue that purgeth cholere, as is sayd in the remedyes foɿ peyne of the head comming of cholere, oɿ let the patient vomite, in gyuinge a sharpe syɿupe of soɿelle, wyth warme water, thã put his fingre in his moth so that he may vompt.

Sycke folkes oftẽ diseased in the sto make, demaundes nothinge elles, but to take awaye the payne, not regardyng the tyme whyle the matter may be puɿ ged by vomiting, glister oɿ other laxes

Also there chaunceth sometyme so great paine and sharpe, that foɿ debily tie of vertu it is good to leaue ẏ cause and stycke to the swaging of ẏ payne
F.v.

The Regyment

wherfore it behoueth to procede in maner folowyng.

Remedye for all paynes of the stomake.

Take cemomil, mellilote, wormwood, mallowes wt theyr rootes, leaues of bayes, parietary and peyryalle, of eche a handesfull, linesed a pound, fenugreke halfe a pounde, anees, and fenell seed, of eche halfe an ounce.

The sayde thynges bruised and well sodden in water, wet therin sponges, and the lycour well pressed out, and applied vnto the stomake, one after another, and warmyng them againe, whē they begynne to cole, swagl all maner paynes of þ stomake. And afterward ye must anoynt the stomake with oyle of dylle and camomylle.

An other remedye.

Take an hogges bladder, and fyll it of þ sayd decoction, and lappe in a linnen cloth, and laye it to the stomake and warme it againe when it is colde.

But

of ſyxe.   Fol. xlvii.

But after ye haue made dyuerſe ſuche applications, ye muſt annointe the ſtomake with the oyle aforeſayde.

Yf the payne be remouyng fro place to place, it ſignifyeth it commeth of ventoſitie. Therfore laye vnto it a bag full of meale, ſalte, and commin dryed togyther.

¶ An other remedye.

Take a ſponefull of hote aſſhes, dewe them wyth good wyne, and couer them with a linnen cloth, ẏ it goe rounde about ẏ ſpoone, and laye it to the ſtomake.

¶ An other remedye.

Take a ſheue of breed metely thycke toſte it, and wete it in hote oyle of camomyll, as hote as it cometh from the ouen, or in oyle of ſpyke, and wrappe it in a lynen, & laye it vppon ẏ payne.

¶ An other remedye.

Put a greate boxynge glaſſe vpon the nauyll, and let it be there .i. houre.

¶ An other remedye for payne
of the ſtomake.

Take

The regyment

Take two drammes of diaciminon, of dianiss, of diagalanga, & drynke it with a lytle good wyne, an houre or .ii. before meate. To drike two ounces of maluesey, w a litle of one of ye sayde electuaries, is very good for such paynes as prede of coldnesse or ventositie

In other remedye.

Take, a dramme of galingale i pouder and gyue it to drynke with a lytle hote wyne, and aboue all thynges for pains of ventositie, a singuler remedye is to drynke a lytle Castor, wyth good wine

In other.

Lyke wyse to drynke two houres before meate thre or foure ounces of the decoction of myntes, anneys seedes, comyne and fyne frankensence,

Also it is good to drynke an electuarie called aromaticū, wherof ye may receyue one lozenge euerye mornynge fastynge.

In other specyall medicyne.

Take halfe an ounce of iuce of mistes,

of lyfe.　　　fol.xlviii.

tes, & two drāmes of þ iuice of worm
wood, l'gnū aloes, & cloues & rilo bal
samū, of eche i poudre halfe a scruple,
all myxt togyther, & dronke warme .ii.
or thre houres before meate, are exce=
dyng profytable.

⁋The lyxt Chapter, of re
medyes for diseases.
of the lyuer.

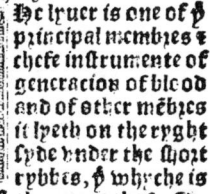

He lyuer is one of þ
principal membres &
chefe instrumente of
generacion of blood
and of other mēbres
it lyeth on the ryght
syde vnder the short
rybbes, þ whyche is
ordeined to digest the meate the secōde
tyme, and thereof to make humours
that nouryssheth all þ membres of mā
nes body, by his naturall heete cōfor
ted by heat of the hert. But somtymes
it is greued by blood into moche aboū
daūce, or by cholerik humours, which
cause to greate heate, or els by fleume
that

The Regiment
that doth diminysh the same.

¶ A remedye for an hote lyuer.

Yf the 'yuer be to hote, bycause of to moch blood, the person hath red vrine hasty pulse, his veines great & full, and he feleth his spattle, mouth and tonge sweter then it was wont to be, wherfore it is good to be let blood of ẏ liuer veine on the ryght arme, and to vse letuse, sorelle, purcelane, and hoppes, in pottage, and sometymes to drynke of the waters of the sayde herbes fasting or els endiue water to refresshe ẏ liuer

¶ Regiment for disease of the liuer comminge of blood.

Ye muste abstaine from drinkynge wine, and eatynge of flesh, and yf at meate or drinke ye must otherwise, the wine ought to be watred, and the fleshe boiled wyth lettuse and sorel. It is better to drynke ptysan, or stale cydre, & eate brothe of peason, almon mylke, hulled barlye, or rosted apples, and damaske prunes, whyles the heate be diminyshed

of lyfe.　　fol.xlix

ſhed. And ye ought euerye daye to pro=
uoke the dutye of the wombe, eyther
by meanes of ſuppoſitorie, or els other
wyſe.

Yf the lyuer be ouer hote by cholere
the pacient hathe hys vryne cleare and
yelowe, without meaſure, great thyrſt
without apperyte, & feleth great bur=
nyng in his bodye, and comonly hath
his bellye bounde, and hathe the face
yelowe.

This diſeaſe of the liuer chaunceth
mooſte in ſomer, & for it ye muſt take
twyſe a daye an ounce of ſyrupe of en=
dyue, or violettes, w a good draught
of ptiſane, drinke it two or thre hou=
res before meate, and alſo at nyght to
bedwarde, and ſo contynue thre or
foure dayes

In ſtede of the ſayd ſyrupes ye may
take thre oſices of ptiſane, or thre oun=
ces of water of endyue, cicorye and ſo=
rell meddled together, for eche tyme.

Then the fyfth daye in the mornynge
early, it is good to drynke a purgaciõ
that

The regiment

that pourgeth cholere, whiche shall be made as foloweth.

¶ An excellent purgation for to auoyde cholere, and maye be gyuen to men of all eges.

Take halfe an ounce of cassia newly drawen, a dtame of good reubarbe infused a nyght in water of endiue with a lytle spikenard and an ounce of syrupe of vyolettes, mixe all the sayde thynges with thre ounces of ptisane or whaye, & drinke it warme as afore is sayd in the other

¶ Boles for the same.

In stede of the said medicine (which is to costlye for poore folkes) ye maye make boles of halfe an ounce of cassia, and thre drammes of electuarium de succo rosarum, and eate them thre houres after mydnyght, and slepe after it, but al the daye ye must kepe ye chamber, & yf ye hed rather drynke it than eate it, mixe the said boles with whay, or endiue water, & drynke it at v. of the clocke in the mornynge, but slepe not after it.

Other

of lyfe.   fol.l.

¶ Other medicines laxatyue.

Talke halfe an ounce of diaprunis laxatyue, myxte with iii. ounces of decoction of french prunes, water of succorie, and drinke it warme at fyue of ye clocke in the mornyng, or els syxe houres afore meate. In steade of the sayde diaprunis, ye maye take halfe an ouce of electuarium de succo rosarum, and make a laxe as afore is sayde.

And it is to be noted, yt the pacyent be very weake or easye to worke vpō, ye maye take away a drame both of the diaprunis & also of succo rosarū. After the said purgation, it is good to refresh the liuer with laying to without on the right syde, vnder the nether ribbes, a playster of cerotum scandalinū, spred vpon a lynnen clothe of ye bygnesse of iiii. fyngers, or bathe the sayd place with a lynnen cloth wet i water of endyue, plantayne and roses, warmed togyther. Moreouer it is good to take euery mornyng before meate a lo-

zenge

zenge of triasandaly, and to drynke after it endyue water. iii. ounces.

❧ Regiment for heate in the lyuer.

The pacient must abstayne from flesh and salt fysh, stronge wyne, garlyke, onyons, mustarde and suche other hote meates. It is good to vse broth of peace with veriuce, lettuce, poppe, spinage, & borage, and sometyme a lytle vynegre yf he be not greued in the stomacke. This regiment is good also in tyme of pestilence, and of to great heate.

❧ A Julep for the heate of the lyuer.

Take halfe a li. of rosewater, one quarter of water of endiue, and v. ounces of sugre, make a iulep, of which ye shal drynke fastyng a good draught. And yf ye wyll nedes drynke for thyrst betwene meales, let it be myngled wyth, ii partes of water of ye wel. And yf ye wyl haue it more colyng, adde vnto it two ounces of vynegre or the iuce of a pomegranade.

Yf the lyuer be colde, for the phlegmatyke

of lyfe. Fol.li.

gmatyke matter that is in it, the persō hath his water white, ¶ out of coloure, the face pale, and his mouth watry, lytele bloode, and feleth heuynesse about hys lyuer.

Remedye.

He ought to drynke in the mornyng earlye. iii. or iiii. tymes a sirupe called oximell diureticum, with the decoction of smalache and perselye, or with waters of smalache, and fenell, and after he must take to purge the fleume a medicyne made as foloweth. Take syxe drammes of diafinicon, if the person be strong, or halfe an ounce if he be weake and distemper it in. iiii. ounces of the decoctiō of thē rootes of smalache, perselye, fenell, and drynke it luke warme v. or. vi. houres afore meate.

In steade of the sayde medicyne one may gyue two drammes of agaryke in troscisbes with water of smalache, or els good fenell.

¶ In other medicine laxatiue.

Take halfe an ounce of diacarthami,

G.ii. or halfe

The regiment.

of halfe an ounce of diapzunis laxatiue oz asmoche of electuarium dulce, with thze ounces of percely water, smallach ysope, oz fenelle, take it fyue houres afoze meate.

☞ Regiment.

The pacient must dzinke good wyne, and vse ginger, cinamome, graynes of paradyse, anyse and fenelle, and hote herbes in pottage, as sage, ysope, tyme maiozym, and auoyde all rawe frutes, and also rawe herbes.

Mozeouer it is verye good to make a playster of smallache, wozmewoodde, spikenarde in pouder, with oyle of dyll myngle it, and lay it vpon the lyuer.

☞ Agaynst stoppyng of the lyuer called oppilation.

Oppilation oz stoppyng cōmeth sometyme in the holownesse of the lyuer, and it is knowen by cō passion and payne of the stomake, and is healed by medicines laxatiue, as it is declared befoze.

And sometyme the oppilation is in the

of lyfe.   Fol.iii.

the veynes of the holowe parte of the lyuer, and is perceyued then by ye grefe which the pacient feleth in his backe, & in his reynes. And it is healed by thinges that open, as by syrupes of the thre rootes, syrupes of bi[?]atius, sirupes of maydenheere, and by drynkyng the decoction of raysins, fenel, percely, smallache, cicorye, or waters stylled of the same herbes. Also rootes of alisaunder is good for the same. &c.

Somtymes the sayd oppilacion cōmeth of grosse blood, carthye, and melancholyke, whiche the membres sende vnto the lyuer, and bycause that suche engendred blood can haue no issue, nor hath any waye to departe to any other membres, therfore be the veynes of the lyuer stopped vp, by the grosnesse of ye sayde bloode. And it is knowen by the water, yt is very hye colour ed, & cleare.

C Remedye.

Gyue the paciēt medicines that perce & subtyle, as is wyne of pomegranates syrupe of endyue, with the decoction of

G.iii.   cicers.

The Regiment

elcers. Then let hym blood on the liuer veyne, and euery mornyng eate a lozēge of triasādaly. Somtyme the sayd oppilacion cōmeth of aboūdaunce of some humour viscouse, colde and flegmatik, stoppynge the veynes of the lyuer, and thē the vrine is as clere as clere water.

⁋ Remedye.

The pacient must drynke euery mornynge the sirupe of orimel squilitike, with half a draught or more of the decoction of rootes of smallache, fenell & percelye. Somtymes vnto women cōmeth oppilations of the lyuer, by reteynyng of theyr purgatiōs. Wherfore it is good to let them blood on the veyne called saphena, whiche is aboue on the hyer syde of the insteppe.

And let them take after the chaunge of the moone seuen or eyght mornynges an opiate called Trifera magna: euerye tyme an ounce. And after drynke thre oūces of waters of mugworte, hysope and fenelle, or the decoction of these herbes, or elles the rootes aperityue,

which

which be smallache, percely, fenell, alisaundre and asperage, boyled in water wyth the thyrde parte of odoriferous whyte wyne.

¶ Medicines for the liuer that may be easely had at all tymes.

Take a good handful of liuerworte that groweth vpon the stones, and another of fumitorye, with as moche of hartestonge, and seeth them in whaye clarifyed, and drynke them euery daye twyse.

The liuer of an hare dryed and made in pouder, is good for all diseases of ye liuer, as affirmeth Auicenne and other of the Arabiens.

Also for heate in the liuer seeth barberyes in wheye, and drynke them.

¶ The .vii. chapter, agaynst the diseases of the galle.

The galle is placed in the holownesse of ye lyuer, to receiue the superfluitie of cholere, & to sende it to the bowels to be auoyded with the grosser excrementes,

¶ The regiment

to thintent to clense the bloode of the sayde cholere.

¶ To the whiche there commeth oftentymes oppilations in the partyes aboute by the lyuer, or beneth in it selfe next the bowels, causyng great payne, by reason wherof the cholere turneth agayne vnto the lyuer, and there is mēgled with the bloode, and spred abrode into all the veynes of the bodye, and bredeth a disease named iaundys (ictericia in latin) wherof be thre kyndes, þ is to saye, yelowe iaundys that procedeth of cholere called citrine or yelowe, grene iaudys which procedeth of grene cholere, and blacke iaundys that procedeth of blacke choler, which is called melancholye, and commonly cōmeth of the oppilation of the splene.

¶ Remedye for iaundys.

Yf the iaundys happen in an ague, before the seuenth daye, the pacyente is in great daunger of his lyfe, as Hipocrates sayeth. But yf it appeare in the syxth daye, being a day iudiciall or cretike

of lyfe. Fo.liiii.

tike of the ague, or after, it is a verye good sygne.

And then ye must succoure nature, in refreshyng and digesting the choler, with sirupe of vyolettes, gyuen in the mornynge with water of morell, or syrupe of endyue, with water of cicorye.

After this, pourge the cholere as is sayd in remedyes of the lyuer: And thā gyue hym a lozenge of triasādali, with reubarbe, euery mornynge two houres before meate, and drynk a lytle waters of endyue, and cicorye, afore the sayde lozenge.

Moreouer, it is good to bathe the lyuer as it is sayde afore, and wach the pacientes eyes wyth vynegre, and womans mylke, and drynk a ptisane made of barly, liquirice, prunes, and the rootes of fenell. And yf (when the feuer is paste) the iaundys taryeth styll, the pacyent must drynke water of fenell, and morelle, with the syrupe of occisaccarū cōpost, and it is good to laye a quycke tenche vpon the liuer.

Iaūdys

The Regiment

Jaundys sometyme commeth withoute feuer, and maye be healed by the thynges that I declared here before, or thus.

In other remedye for the Jaundys.

Take foure ounces of radysshe, and gyue it the sycke to drynke. v. mornynges thre houres afore meate. In steade wherof it is good to drynke euery mornynge foure ounces of the decoction of horehounde, made in whyte wyne, or as moche of the decoction of celydonye and barberyes, wyth a lytle honye and saffron.

In other remedye.

Take wormes of the earth called angle twiches, and wash them i white wyne, then drye them and drynke them a spooncful at a tyme, ī whyte wyne.

In other.

Ye maye let hym drynke. vii. or. viii. dayes togyther ī þ mornynges, a good draught of the decoction of politrichō, or of maydenheere. The decoction also of of lyfe. fol.lv.

of woodbynde, or the water of it distilled in a common stylle, is a soueraygne
medicine for the sayde disease.

℄ An other singuler
remedye.

Take cowes mylke and whyte wyne
of eche a pynt, and distill them in a still
kepe that water a moneth, and then
gyue it to the pacient thre ounces in the
mornyng two houres afore meate, and
lykewyse after supper, when he goeth
to bedde.

℄ The eyght Chapter, for
diseases of the splene.

The splene is a membre lõge
softe, and spongy, beinge
in ye lefte syde ioyned vnto the holownesse of ye stomacke, and to the thycke
endes of ye rybbes, & to ye
backe, the whiche is ordeyned for to receyue the melancholy humours, & to cle-
anse the blood of the same, for by that
meane ye blood remayneth pure & nette.
Wherfore it is good nourishyng for al
the

the membres, and is the cause that maketh a bodye merye, but oftentymes there happeneth oppilatiō or debilitie wherof commeth the blacke iaundys.

And somtymes it is greater, fuller, or grosser then it ought to be, by ouermuche melancholie that is not natural, caused of the dregges of the blood engendred in the lyuer, & doth hyndre generacion of good blood, wherethrough the membres become drye, for defaute of good nourishynge. And therfore the pacient is called splenetyke, whiche ye maye knowe by that, that after meate they haue payne in theyr left syde, and are alwayes heuye, and hath theyr faces somwhat enclynyng vnto blaknesse

⁋ Remedye.

In oppilacions and apostemes of the splene, whether it be of hote humours or of colde, he ought to be let bloode on ye splene veyne called saluatella, which is in the lefte hande, betwene the lytle fynger, and the next finger which they call medicus. And ye must drawe oute
but

but a lytle blood

And yf the pacient feele a burnynge on the left syde, and hath a drye tonge wythoute appetyte, it signifyeth that suche disease of the splene, is caused of an hote humoure. Wherfore ye muste gyue the paciēt foure or. v. mornynges fastynge, syrupe of endyue water, and hartestōge, then a purgation made as foloweth thus.

⁂ A goodlye purgation to auoyde melancholye.

Take halfe an ounce of succorosarū and thre ounces of the decoction of the rootes of capparus, and hartestonge, & make a drynke the whiche ye may mynystre in a good day to take purgatiōs syxe houres afore meate.

⁂ An other.

In stede of that drynke ye may tempre halfe an ounce of cassia, and thre drammes of diasenye in thre ounces of wheye, or hartestonge water, & drynke it as is aforesayde. After the sayd purgation, ye ought to annoynt the splene
with

The regyment

with oyle of violettes, or oyle of lyne seed, or to make a playster of the sayde oyle and lyneseede, and the rootes of capparis, and laye vpon the splene.

Also after the sayde purgation, it shall be good to laye vppon the splene, nyghtshade, purcelane seede, and pouder of plantayne, nypete with vynegre lyke a playster, and yf the pacient haue more appetyte then he can digeste, and that he haue belchynges of the stomak somtymes soure in the mouth, it signifyeth that the passion splenetike commeth by a colde humour melancholike.

Remedye.

Ye must drynke sirupe of sticados, or harteftonge, or oximel diureticū, with water of the decoction of hartestonge, epythime, smallache rotes, perecly rotes, tameriscus, and myntes, or els one lye wyth the decoction of hartestonge, and rootes of cappars. And then after purge it frō such melancholy humour, wyth an ounce of diacatholicon, & two drames of diasene, dissolued in, iii, ounces of

of lyfe. Fol.lvii.

ees of the sayde decoction, or water of wormewood, or hartestonge.

And after this ye must annoynt the syde of the splene, with oyle of lillyes, oyle of dylle, fresshe butter, marye of an oxe, and hennes grece, or of a dogge, medled togyther, or annoynt the sayde syde wyth dialthea

And ye pacient ought to drinke white wine, and the decoction of hartestong, euenynge and mornynge, takynge two fygges, wyth pouder of ysope, pepper or gynger, but he maye put no water in hys wyne, and oftentimes he must eate cappars, with a lytle oyle and vinegre.

If for the oppilations of the splene, the pacient hath a pa e colour, or leady in the face, and a whytenes of eyes, takynge awaye of appetite, payne in the lefte syde wyth hardenesse, and hathe hys excrementes blacke, it is a signe of the blacke iaundys.

⁋An expert medecine for all diseases of the splene.

Take the leaues and coddes of seny
the

The regyment

the barke of an asshe tre skraped & cutte maydenheare, hartestõg and liquirice, seeth them all in clere whaye and after they be strayned drynke of it twyes or thryes a daye tyl ye be amended.

¶ Remedye for the blacke
iaundys,

Ye muste gyue syrupes & purgations as afore is sayde, and to be let blood of the veyne saluatella, and afterwarde diuers tymes euenynge and mornyng, to apply vētoses vpon the splene without scarifyinge. Afterwarde ye muste lay on it a liste, wette in good vinegre, and kepe it there so longe as the heate remayneth in the sayde lyste, & warme it thre or foure tymes.

Afterwarde annoynt the splene with dialthea, and so contynew four or fiue dayes, and other foure or fyue dayes lay vpon it a plaister made of two oũces of gumme armoniake dissolued in vinegre, aud spred vpon lether.

And yf by the forsayde thynges the pacient be not eased, the doctours of
physycke

of lyfe.   Fol. lxvi.

phisycke saye, that he must receyue the medicines agayne, at the leste ones in euery moneth, for halfe a yere togither.

⁋ Regiment for al
oppilacions.

The pacient ought to vse thynges of easye digestion, and in smal quantitie, and ought to absteyne from breade to lytle leuened, cakes, tartes, pastyes, pyes, hogges fleshe, beafe, and poudred meates, and fumyshe. Fishe, lymmons, peason, beanes mylke, chese, ryse, and firmentie, al fryed meates, drynke after supper, wyne and apples, whyche wyth al other lyke trouble the bodye. Also ye must absteyne from muche mouyng or exercise by and by after meate.

It is good to vse capars, asparage, hoppes, brothe of dryed peason, wyth perceley or hys rotes, smal byrdes of the felde, kyddes fleshe, yonge mutton, lambe, chyckyns, feysauntes, snytes, partriches, scaled fyshe, of swete runnynge water, wyth perceley and vinegre. Newe layed egges potched in wa-

.H.   ter,

The Regiment

ter, are verye holsome, & ye may drynke whyte wyne or claret, onely at meales.

Also it is good to vse cresses, sage, ysope, myntes, fenel, and percely, succorye, scariole, and beetes, and singulerlye, to take fastyng halfe a sponekfull of redde colewortes sodden, & to eate often anyse seedes, and fenel.

¶ The nynth Chapter, for diseases of the bowelles.

In a person be sixe guttes. iii. smal, whyche are situate ouer ye nauylle, & .iii. greate, whyche are placed vnder the nauyl.

The fyrst is called duodenum, bycause it is .xii. ynches longe.

The seconde is called ieiunum, for that nothyng remayneth in it.

The thyrde is called ylis, bycause it is longe and smal.

The fourth which is ye fyrst of ye great ones, is called monoculus, bicause it is lyke a sacke, & hath but one mouth & in that same sometymes are wormes engendred of lyfe.   Fo.lxi.

engendred or ventosite, that causeth peyne of the bellye on the ryght syde, whyche is not the very colycke.

¶The.v.they cal colon, bicause it hath many holowe places, and it procedeth from the ryght syde vnder the lyuer, & it maketh hys reuolucyon vnto the left syde, wherein is engendred the colyke whyche is dispersed by all the bellye, more then any other disease.

¶The.vi. is called rectum, bycause it is nye vnto the left kydneye, and goeth euen ryght downe into the foūdament.

Hipocrates calleth the thre bowelles that are nexte the stomake plia, that is to saye smal guttes, & the peyne of one of them is called pliaca passio, a verye sharpe peyne. Rasis calleth it, domine miserere. & ykewyse also colica passio, is called of the gutte colon, whyche. ii. diseases are sisters, for asmoch as they come oftentimes both of one cause, that is to say of ye oppylation of ye bowelles

¶Remedye for the collicke
and of pliaca passio.
H.ii.   Foras-

The regyment

Forasmuche as those diseases are excedynge egre, sharp, and almooste importable of peyne, wherof many tymes foloweth defection of the strength, wyth varietie of medicines ye ought incontinentlye for to helpe them.

Fyrste when the sayde peynes come by the stoppynge of the bellye, ye muste gyue him a glister mollificatyue, made of the decoctiõ of mallowes, violettes, beetes, anyse seed and fenugreke, with cassia, and comon honye, and oyle olyue, and afterwarde, the herbes of the sayd glister brused & fryed, & layed hote betwixt .ii. linins, & applied to the belly.

And yf by thys meanes the peyne cease not, let the patient sytte vnto the buttockes, in the sayde decoction, and after wyth dialthea & butter, annoynte thy nauyl.

And if the sayd glyster do not worke sufficiently, make another of the same, or els gyue hym a suppositorye whych is longe ynough, made of pure honye,
and

of lyfe. fol.lxiiii.

and sal gemme.

⸿ For the wyndye collyke.

Thorow wyndines oftentymes, cōmeth the colica passio, or iliaca, & then it appeareth that the peyne is chaūgeable, and mouyng from place to place, and is knowen also by the romblynge which is a noyse in the bowelles, with gryppynges, and great peyne.

⸿ Remedye.

Take mallowes, beetes, & mercury of eche a good handful, margerim, & uc, bayes, and camomyl, of eche a lytle handeful, anyse seedes, comyn, of eche an ounce, make a decoctiō, & take therof a pynt and a halfe, and dissolue in it an ounce of cassia, halfe an ounce of triacle and .iii. oūces of oyle olyue or of camomyl, & make a glyster, the whych must be gyuen warme vnto the patient, long before or after meate.

In sted of the sayde glyster, ye may gyue hym a pounde of oyle of lineseede, whyche is a singuler thynge to take awaye al diseases of the belly. Also it is

H.iii. good

The regiment

good to make a myxture wyth oyle of hempe seed.

⟪ For to appease the peyne caused of wynde.

Fyrste make a glyster of maluesaye, oyle of camomyl, or dyl. If for the sayd glysters the peyne cease not, or els the pacient wyl not take them, take a great sponge or els a felt of a hatte, and stepe it in wine of the decoction of rue, camomyl, maiorym, anyse seedes, and commyn. And afterwarde laye it vpon the peyne, as hote as the patient can suffre, and .iiii. tymes in the daye, it is good to let hym drynke wyne wherin hath bene sodden rue seedes, careawayes, and commyne. Drynke at euerye tyme a lytle draught, and eche daye kepe abstinence from eatynge and drynkynge moche of other thynges tyl ye be perfectly hole.

⟪ A suppository for the wyndye colyke.

Take a dramme of rue in fyne pouder and halfe a drame of commyne dryed and poudred, and wyth honye skūmed,

make

of lyfe. fol. lxl.

make a suppository.

℃ A playster for wyndye colycke.

Take two handfulles of rue, in fine
pouder, myrre, and compne poudred of
eche halfe an ounce, four egges yolkes,
and make two playsters wyth honye,
and laye on the one at nyght, and the other in the mornynge, vpon the bellye.
Water of camomyl, or a decoction of
the same droken, is good for them that
haue such diseases. Also a dryed acorne
in pouder, and gyuen to drynke wyth
whyte wyne, is very good.

If ye knowe that the peyne of the
bellye commeth thorough wynde, applie vpon it a greate ventose wythout
incisyon, for by that meanes the sayde
peyne wyl surelye go a waye, or dyminysshe. If not, it sheweth that there is
some humours that causeth the sayde
peyne, as fleume or cholere.

If by fleume it commeth, ye muste
make a glister of a pynte of the decoction of camomil, rue, wormewood, maio
H.iiii. rum,

The regyment.

rim, mellilote, centaurie, anise seedes, and fenel, and in the same decoction put halfe an ounce of heira picra, or halfe an ounce of diafinicon, and .iii. ounces of oyle of dil, or of lillies.

Also ye ought to giue to the pacient sirupe of wormwood, and to make application vpon his bellie as hathe bene sayde afore, or to laye vnto it gromell seed & baye salt dryed togither, whiche layed vpon the bellie, is lykewise good for the wyndye collicke.

If after the sayde thinges the sayde peyne continueth, ye muste make a purgation as foloweth.

A purgation for colike commynge of fleume.

Take. v. drammes of diafinicon, iii. ounces of wormewood water, & make a drynke, the whyche receyued fasting, iiii. or. v, houres afore meat, is verye profitable.

For peyne of the colicke commynge of choler.

If the sayde peyne cometh of choler,

of lyfe.　　　Fol.lxit.

ler, whiche is knowen when by the application of hote thinges the peyne encreaseth, ye must make a glister of violets, or giue him halfe an ounce of succo rosarū w^t ptisan, endiue water or wine

And the next mornyng let him drinke a ptisane of the decoctiō of prunes, and violet floures, and annoynt the belly wyth oyle of violettes, or wette a lynnē cloth ī colde water & laye it thervpō.

If it do continew styl, the patient must be sette in warme water vp to the hanches, and yf the peyne come of cold, ye must annoynt his belly with oyle of bayes, and gosegrese.

⁋ For the wyndy colycke.

If it be winde, make a glister of new mylke wyth a lytle oyle, and the yolke of an egge, for it is very good. Also it is good to lette hym drynke a dramme of hiera picra simpler, wyth .ii. ounces of water of cardo benedictus, or purcelane or wormewood, and to make a playster of lecke leaues fryed in oyle and vinegre, and layed vpon the bellye.

　　　　　H.v.　　　Lyke-

The Regyment

Lykewyse it is good to drynke the iuyce of enula campana, or the sirupe therof, & to were a playster vpon ye bellie, made of hony, wormewood & aloes.

¶ A glyster for al colicke.

Take the oldest cocke ye can gette, the whyche muste be wel beaten wyth smal roddes, and then chop of the head and put in a good sufficiencie of water, and scalde hym, and trymme hym for to seeth. And wyth in the bellye of the sayde cocke put anyse seedes, fenel, compn, polipody, and the seedes of cartami, of eche halfe an ounce, turbith, sene, and agaryke, bounde surelye in a lynnen clothe, of eche two drammes, floures of camomyl an handeful, seeth them vntyl the flesh go from the bones and take of the said decoction a pound, and a quartron of oyle of camomyl, and dyl, and thre or foure ounces of egge-yolkes, make a glyster whyche must be gyuen warme, longe before or after meate, or drynke.

Pillule cochie are very good for the sayde

of lyfe. Fol. lxiii.

sayde disease, speciallye when the glyster doth not suffice, to purge the cause of the same. Also diamasci, and diaciminum are very good lectuaryes, yf ye take of one of them a lozenge fastynge, two houres before meate. Lykewyse it is good to take mithridatum, with a lyttle whyte wyne, or wyth the decoction of camomyl, foure or fyue houres after dynner, yf hys belly be naturally laxe, or els by some suppositorye or glyster.

¶ Against disease of the raynes of the backe, and the loynes.

PAyne of the reynes is called nephritica passio, & cōmeth of some one or grauel, & it is most lyke vnto the colicke in cure, but in causes they be cleane contrarie: for the colicke begynneth at the lower partes on the righte side, and goeth vp to the hyer partes on the left side, of the belly, and it lyeth rather more forwarde then backewarde, but nephritica passio begynneth contrarywise aboue, descendyng downewarde, and euer lieth more towarde

The regyment
warde the backe.

Also nephretica is paynfuller afore meat, and the colicke is euer more greuous after. And often the colicke chaūceth sodenlie, but nephretica contrarie, for commonlie it commeth by litle and litle, for euermore before, one shal fele payne of ẏ backe w difficultie of vrine.

Item there is more difference, for the colicke sheweth vrynes as it were coloured, but nephretica in the begynuinge is cleare, and white like water, & after waxeth thycke, and then appeareth in the botome of the vessel leke red sande or grauel.

⁋ Remedie for peyne of
the reynes

Ye must vse thinges aperitiue, to cause you make water, but afore ye ought to lose the belly in taking an ounce of cassia, an houre before meate, but if your bellie be harde bounde, ye must take a glister made as hereafter foloweth, before ye take the sayde cassia.

A glister

A glister for nephre-
tica passio.

Take of marche mallowe rotes two ounces, mallowes, violettes, beetes, and marche mallowe leaues, floures of camomylle and mellilote, of eche a handeful, melon seede and anyse seed, of eche halfe an ounce, wheate branne, an handful, and decocte it, and take therof halfe a pounde, and distemper in it an ounce of cassia, & an ounce of course suger. ii. ounces of oyle of violettes, & an ounce of oyle of lilies, make a glyster. In stede therof ye may take cowes mylke, with two egge yolkes, in maner of a glyster.

And it is to be noted, that in suche a disease, the glystre muste be greate in quantitie, or els ye shulde make wrestynge & roumblynge in ye bellye, whiche shulde be an occasyon of more payne,

After this operation, if the payne be not apeased, ye must gyue another glyster after the operation of whyche, the patient ought to go into some bath, vp
to the

to the naupl, wherein muste be sodden mallowes, marche mallowes, beetes, pellitarye, lyneseed, fenugreke, & floures of camomyl, wyth mellilote, al put in a bagge in the sayd water, and rubbe hym wyth it, and at hys goynge out of the sayd bath, ye must take two ounces of sirupe of mayden heare, & radishe, w iii. ounces of þ decoction of lyquiriec. Moreouer after the sayde bath, ye must laye vppon the payne a pultes made of herbes, and floures, with oyle of almōdes, beyng in the sayde bagge, and. ii. or iii. morninges take. v. or. vi. ounces of þ brothe of cicers, sodden wyth lycorice, or els drink water of pellitory, of cresses, or of rotes aperitiue, the which waters are verye good, for to purge þ grauel and the stone.

Lykewyse a very good electuary for the same, called electuarium ducis, or iustinum, philantropos, or liontripon, yf one take a dramme or two after operation of a glister, or of cassia, or a pylle of ante cibū, and after to drynke one of
the

of lyfe. Fol.lxv.

the sayde waters, or elles a litle whyte wyne warmed.

¶ Regiment aswel for the colyke, as for the reynes of the backe.

HE must flye from al euyll qualities of the ayre, as wynde, rayne, great heate, and greate colde, specyallye to kepe him from warmyng the reynes agaynst the fyre, nor to heat it by any other meanes. Also he muste abstayne from great repletion at one meale, and to longe abstinence from meate, for all these fille the bodie ful of yll humours. Also sleape not on the daye, specially after meate, nor lye not on the reynes, when ye are aslepe.

And ye ought to eate no saltfysh, nor no byefe, nor other grosse meates. Lyke wise one ought for to beware of al foules bredde vp in the water, spycery, pastrye, and bread not verye well leuened specially tartes, cakes, and other pasties made of flour. But aboue al, ye must beware of whitemetes, as milke, chese

rawe

The Regyment.

aw e fr utes, harde egges, & as moch as is possible, kepe your selfe frõ yre, enuye, melancholy, & other lyke affectiõs.

¶ For the flure of the wombe.

IN al fluxes of ý belly, cause the excremẽtes to be dulye serched, for if the disease be suche, that the meate commeth out, euen as it was receyued, or not half dygested, ý sayde flure is called lienteria. Yf great aboundaũce of waterye humours haue theyr issue by lowe, the sayde flure is named diarrhea, whyche is as moch to saye as flure humorall. And yf bloode or matter appeare wyth the excrementes in the syckenesse, then they call it dissenteria, which is a gret disease and a daungerous for to cure.

¶ Remedy for the flure lienteria.

FOrasmoch as this flur cõmeth for the most parte of great debilitie of vertue retentyue of the stomacke, for ý great moystnes of the same, it is good to gyue ý sirupe of wormewood, and honye of roses, taking kyng of it with a spone, or drynke the wyth the water of betonye, fenell, and wormewood, and yf it so be the paciente doo desyre to vomyte, it wolde be good for hym, or let hym take halfe an ounce of hiera simple, wyth two ounces of water of wormewood, and if the pacient be stronge ynough, adde therto two drammes of diafinicon.

And after thys ye muste comforte the stomake with oyle of mastyke, spike, mynt, wormewood, or nardine, or with a playstre called cerotum Galeni, spred vpon lether, and after layed vppon the stomacke, or make a bagge of wormewood, myntes, and maiorim dryed, and laye it vpon the stomake.

In the mornynge take a lozenge of aromaticum rosatum, and a lytle rynde of citron cōfit, and before euery meale take a morcel of conserua quynces.

☞ Remedye for the fluxe humoral called diarthea.

The sayde fluxe oughte not to be restrayned afore the .xiiii. daye, yf na-

The regyment.

ture be not very moch enfebled. And somtyme it commeth of hote causes, as of cholere, and thē one oughte to gyue vnto the paciente to drynke afore his meate syrupe of ribes, syrupe of roses, or syrupe of quinces, wyth smythes water, and ī the stede of those syrupes, ye may make a iulep thus.

A iulep for the fluxe humorall.

Take rosewater, buglosse, and plantayne, euerye one halfe a pounde, of all the saunders two drammes, and wyth a quartron and an halfe of sugre, make a iulep. In the mornyng two houres afore meat, it is good to gyue the paciēt olde conserue of roses, or a dramme of troeiskes of roses after he hath dronke one of the sayde syrupes, or of iulep of roses wyth a lytle of smythes water, wherof the pacient ought to drynke at euery tyme whē he is a thyrst.

Yf in the sayde fluxe there be egre matter, and the strength of the pacient any thynge constaunt, ye maye minister the

laua=

of lyfe.   Fol. lxvii.

lauatorie that hereafter enſueth.
¶ Take redde roſes, barly, plantayne, of euery one a handfull, ſeth them, and in the ſtreynyng. adde. ii. ouces of oyle of roſes, one ounce of honye of roſes, and the yolke of an egge, and gyue it in the maner of a gliſter.

Sometyme it is expedient to take a medicine by the mouthe, and it is made as thus.

¶ A medicine for the fluxe.
¶ Take the ryndes of myrabolane citrine baken one dramme, reubarbe a lytle dryed vppon a tyle, halfe a dramme, ſyrupe of quinces one ounce, water of plantayne. iii. ounces, myngle al togyther, and lette the pacient drynke them foure houres before meate, & than giue hym a glyſter retentyue made as thus.

¶ A glyſter for the fluxe.
¶ Take oyle of roſes, of quinces of maſtike, ofeuery one thre ouces, bole armonyak in pouder. ii. drammes, meddle al togyther and gyue it as a glyſter.

¶ An other,

J ii.   Take

The regymment

Take the iuce of plantayne, of popy of bursa pastoris, and oyle of quinces, of euerye one .iii. ounces, myngle them togyther, and gyue it for a glyster. And if the bowels be excoriate, ye shall giue this peculier remedye. Take halfe one pounde of mylke, the water wherein gaddes of stele hath ben quenched, the iuce of plantayne, and oyle of quinces, of euerye one .ii. ounces, bole armenye on dramme, goates tallowe one ounce, and make them in a glyster, but wythout vppon the stomacke, ye muste laye thys oyntmente that here foloweth.

An oyntment for the fluxe.

Take oyles of roses, quinces, & mirtilles, of eche an ounce, oyle of mastyk, halfe an ounce, pouder of coral, and nuttes of cipresse, of euerye one a dramme, myngle all wyth ware, and make an oyntment. Here is to be noted that the glisters that are gyuen for to stoppe a fluxe, must be verye lytle in quantitie.

Ye maye heale the fluxe of dissenteria with gyuynge thynges before declared
for

of lyfe. Fo.lxviii.

foꝛ the fluxe humoꝛall, and take afoꝛe your repast.ii.dꝛammes of conserue of quinces,oꝛ of marmelade of quinces. And he ought to dꝛynke water, wherin hath ben quenched gaddes of stele, and ye muste auoyde diuersitie of meates, and gyue your selfe to ease,and to quyet, and slcape a great whyle. And it is good to vse grewel,clene barlye, and almon mylke, wyth a lytle amidum, and set ventoses vpon the bellye withoute cuttyng, whiche thinge is also good in al fluxes of the body. If the sayde flux humoꝛal pꝛocedeth of fleume,it shal appeare of the excrementes that are watrye and flegmatyke, & than ye oughte to gyue.iii.oꝛ.iiii.moꝛninges, syꝛupe of woꝛme wood, oꝛ of mynte, after purgation as is here folowynge.

¶ A purgation foꝛ the flux humoꝛal.

Take.ii.dꝛames of mirabolanes dꝛied on a tile, halfe a scrupule of agarike in trociske, halfe an ounce of sirupe of mynte,oꝛ.ii.ouces of water of bawme

J.iii. and

and make a potion that shall be receyued .iii. or .iiii. dayes, aftre meate.

If ye wyll make a iulep, take water of mynte, and of bawme, of euerye one halfe a pounde, suger a quarterne, and make a iulep, of the whyche one maye drynke euenyng & mornyng after meat euery tyme a draught. Euery mornyng it is good to take a lozenge of the elecctuarie that foloweth.

A noble electuarye for the fluxe.

Take pouder of diagalanga a dramme and a halfe, of redde coral and mastike, of euery one a scruple, trociskes of terra sigillata half a dramme, the barkes of citrons comfyt, and quinces, of euery one thre drammes, suger dyssolued in water of myntes, foure ouces, make an electuarye.

Oyles of wormewood, mynte and of narde, and mastyke, are verye holsome to annoynt wythal the bellye, & the stomake, for the sayde fluxe.

And the thynges declared of the fluxe lienteria,

lienteria, be verye good in this case, ta=
kyng euer after meate, a morsel of mar=
malade. Redde wyne is verye good in
this fluxe, to drynke at meate wyth the
water of a smyth, and lykewyse all
spices are good for the same
purpose.

℘ Medicines to restrayne the
fluxe, of whatsoeuer
cause it be.

Ake the pesyll of an harte, and
drye it into pouder, & drinke it.
The water of oken buddes,
or the verye acornes dryed and
made in pouder, and dronken in redde
wyne, is verye good.
Item the mawe of a yonge leue=
rette, wyth the iuyce of
playntayne is exce
dynge profy=
table.

℘ The tenth chapter, of
diseases of the
matryce.
J.iiii. Fi℞st

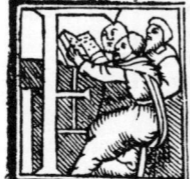

The regiment

Yrst agaynst superfluous fluxe of the mother, in ẏ whyche ye must cōsydre whether it doo come of to greate quantitye of bloode, and then it is good for to open the veyne saphena, and abstayne frō al thynges that multiplye the bloode, as egges, wyne and flesshe. Or whether it cōmeth of cholere, and then ye must receyue a lytle syrupe of roses, pomegranades, or ribes with water of plātayn. Thā purge the choler that gyueth such sharpenesse to the bloode, by ten drammes of trifera sarracenica, with .ii. ounces of plantayne water, or the medicine of reubarbe, wrytten in the treatyse of the fluxe humorall.

After purgation ye maye gyue euery mornyng a lozenge of triasandali, or a dramme of trosciskes of roses, in pouder, after drynke two ounces of plantayne water. And yf suche fluxe of the matrice,

matrice, happen of the watrynesse of blood, gyue her to drynke .iiii. or .v. mornynges, hony of roses wyth a litle water of wormewoode, afterwarde purge her wyth a dr̄ame and a halfe of agarik in troscifkes, and halfe an ounce of trifera sarasenica, myxte wyth water of minte, and of wormewood.

Ye may knowe the causes of the sayd fluxe, by annoyntyng a threde or cloute in the sayde blood, for if it hath the coloure of vermylon, it sygnyfyeth that the fluxe cōmeth of to moche blood. If it appere a lytle yelowe, it signifyeth that the dysease commeth of the subtilitie & sharpnes of the blood, ouercome wyth choler. And if it hath a coloure lyke the water in whiche newe flesshe is wasshed, it betokeneth the blood is moch watrye.

And after ye haue purged the principall cause of the disease, youre seconde intention shalbe, by and by to staunche the said yssue. Wherin also one thinge is to be noted, that if nature be accustomed

The regyment

med to auoyd any superfluytes, by cõtynual course of the sayd fluxe, it wold perchaunce be inconuenient for to stop it, wherfore yf ye se no ieoperdye, ye maye restrayne the sayd flux this wise.

¶ Remedye for to stoppe the sayde fluxe.

¶ Take troscisches of white amber, and make them in pouder, and gyue a drame cuery mornynge, and anon after, drink an ounce, or .ii. of water of plantayne.

In steade of these trociskes, ye maye make a poudre of sãguis draconis, bole armeny, whyte ambre, and redde coral, drynkynge one dramme thereof, wyth plantayne water as is aforesayde.

¶ An other medecine to staunch the sayde fluxe.

¶ Take two ounces of olde conserue of roses, of the sede of plantayne .ii. drammes, sanguinis draconis, bole armeny, of cuerye one a drãme & an halfe, whyte coral and redde, ana one dramme, make a confection with sirupe of myrtilles, & gyue it to drynke, mornynge & euenyng

two

ii.houres afore meate, at euerye tyme
the quantitie of a meane chesnutte.

⁜ For the same.

Applye ventoses vnder the breastes,
twyse a daye, before dynner and sup=
per, and vse to beare about your necke,
or holde alwayes in your hande, redde
corall, iaspys, or a stone called hemati=
tes, whyche is a singuler remedye for
to stoppe euerye kynde of bloodye flux=
es, yf it be borne, or tempered in wyne
and dronke, or make thereof a pouder,
and vse of it euery mornyng with a ly=
tle wyne.

⁜ For reteynyng of the floures.

Sometymes there chaũceth vnto wo=
men when they can not haue theyr due
purgations, to fal in greuous kyndes
of sycknesses, for the auoydaũce where=
of, it is good to helpe thẽ, and prouoke
the sayde purgations by suche thyn=
ges as open, whyche muste be gyuen
at suche tyme of the moone, as the sayd
women were wont to haue the same.

And yf ye se the womans bloode to
be to

The regyment

be to grosse and thycke, so that she can not haue anye such purgation, ye must euerye moneth gyue her the syrupe of fumetorye, wyth the decoction of borage, and buglosse, and let her bathe her selfe, wyth fresshe water, hoote.

And when she goeth out of the bath in to the bedde, she muste receyue the forsayd syrupe and decoction of the herbe called rubea tinctorum or madder, sodden in cleare water. In stede of syrupes ye maye take the verye iuyce or decoction of the herbes.

And if the womans blood be slympe, colde, & flegmatyke, then she must drinke sirupe of sticados, & of oximel diuretike and afterwarde take the pylles called fetide, and of agaryke. And euery mornynge after that, she must take a drame of troscisskes de mirrha, with two ounces of the decoction of Juniper beries, or two drammes of trifera magna and therupon drynke two ounces of water of Mugworte.

And yf perchaunce ye can not haue these

these thynges at nede, ye may take .iii. ounces of the decoction of alisaunders the roote of smallache, cinamome, and a lytle saffron, and let her drynke therof two tymes a daye, and eate no meat therafter, duryng foure houres.

Moreouer it is a proued and expert medicyne, to giue the first day of ye new moone a dramme of poudre made of borax, which the goldesmithes do occupy wyth asmoche cynamome, and a lytle water of smallach. Also it is very good to haue the veyne opened, whych is called saphena, that lyeth outewarde betwene the insteppe and the heele.

And yf case so be, that the said retention come of superfluitie, or to moch aboundaunce of fatte, then the chefe remedie is to suffre moche hunger, and to eate very lytle, moche excercyse and labour, to prouoke swete, and to slepe as lytle as maye be possyble

But yf it come of greate debilitye & weakenes of the bodye, when the natural strengthe is ouercome by reason of
some

The regyment

some sykneſſe, or after a longe ague, in thys caſe ye maye not go about to prouoke the ſayde purgation, but wyth al your endeuoure ſeke to reſtore nature, and gyue the pacient thynges of moche nouryſhment, as potched egges, good fleſhe and good wyne, with other lyke.

Sometyme the ſayde retention commeth of the exceſſyue heate of nature, in ſome women, ſpecyallye ſuche as be valyaunt and ſtrōge as men, and thoſe that are wont to moche labour, by reaſon whereof the heate of theyr bodyes is ſo ſtrōge, that they nede none of the ſayde purgations, for the ſuperfluities of theyr bodyes, are ſufficientlye conſumed of the heate alone, therfore they haue no nede of the ſayde remedyes.

⁋ For chokynge or ſuffocation of the matrice.

The matrice or mother in a woman, oftentymes mounteth vp, towarde the midreſe and the ſtomcke, wyth intollerable paynes, and is called, ſuffocation, bycauſe that it is choked, or ouercharged of lyfe.   Fol.lxxiii.

chaunged wyth some cuyll and superfluous matter, as by stoppynge of the due purgations, or to moche abstinence of Venus, wherby is often chaunced shortnesse of breath, payne of the head, swownynge, tremblynge of the hearte contraction of membres, and otherwhyles death wythout remedye.

¶ A medicine for the said disease.

Ye must rubbe the legges and wrestes of the armes vehementlye, & bynd them with cordes or with garters, tyll they waxe sore, then set ventoses vpon the legges, and al to chafe the stomacke specially beneth round about the nauil.

And then ye muste constrayne her to smell stynkyng thynges as assa fetida, galbanū, pertryche fethers brente, and the quenchinge out of candels, with other suche, but byneth ye muste applye thynges of swete odoure, as gylofloures, maioram, lignum aloes, ambre, cyuet, and a trosciske of gallia muscata, & let her drynke a draught of thys recept,

that

The regiment,
that foloweth.
¶ A drynke for payne of
the mother.

Take one dramme of mithridatum, and dissolue it in an ounce and an halfe of water of wormewood, and giue it to her to drynke, afore she go to meate. iiii houres.

¶ Dyuers goodly medicines for diseases of the mother what soeuer be the cause.

Take the rasing of yuery and the rasyng of an hartes horne with the heare of an hare, dryed and made in pouder, and asmoche of gotes clawes brēt and poudered yf they maye be gotten, or in steade of it shepes clawes, take al these and vse to eate them in youre potage or otherwyse, to stoppe the fluxes of the matrice.

¶ An other to prouoke them.

Sethe marygoldes, nepte and sauine in good ale, and drynke it wyth a good quantitye of saffron, and a lytle honye or suger.

Item

of lyfe. fol. lxxv

Item .xv. blacke seedes of pionie, dronken in wyne wyth saffron, purgeth the matrice of humours, and other. xv. of the redde seedes, staūcheth it agayne, or any other fluxe of the mother.

¶ An other.

These herbes are good to purge the matrice, Rue, peony, saupne, betonye, nepte, valerian, maydenheare, horehounde, sauery, percely, gromel alysaunder, marigoldes, smallache, and tyme.

¶ The .xi. Chapter, of the cure of the stone in the reynes, and in the bladder.

Pyne of the stone is one of the most enormous paynes that the bodie of man is vexed with, for by it many tymes the natural vertues are distroyed, women lose their frute afore the time, cruel & perillous accidentes commonlye do encrease, yea and oftentymes death without remedie.

R.i. Whē

The Regiment

Wherfore it shalbe expedient to the conforte of the poore folkes, and other that be greued, to write some good and holesome medicines for auoydynge of the stone.

¶ And seynge that al authours do affirme the stone to be engēdred by reason of the great heat that is about the reynes, streytnesse of the condites, and aboūdaūce of grosse & slymye fleume, or of brent choler, which by ye sayd excesse of heate, is as one wolde saye, baken or dryed as claye is in the furneys, and so at last becommeth an harde stone, therfore it is chefely to be noted, that without amendyng of the foresayde causes, all that ye do ministre for to breake the stone is eyther hurtful to the patient, or els of smal effecte. For the which cause it is very necessary that ye patient kepe a sobre diete.

And for the better vnderstandynge, ye shall know, that al wynes (whether they be swete or sharpe, grosse or subtyl, whyte or redde) are in this case vtterlye

terlye reiected.

Pulses also of what kynde soeuer they be, as pease, beanes, and such, and al grosse flesshe, and water foules, and foules of greate bodies, as bustardes, cranes, and suche lyke, are in this case very daungerous and noysome.

Also ye maye eate no kynde of frutes, excepte it be a fewe melons, rype prunes in smal quantitie, & pomgranades, with a lytle sugre and coriandres.

Of herbes, ye maye eate borage, buglosse, percely, lettuse, mintes, spinache and succorrye in brothe of veale, or of a yonge chyckyn. Nepes also & rapes, and radysshe, in a smal quantitie, maye be wel ynough permitted.

Potched egges are very good in this case, with a litle vergeouce, but in anye wyse beware of harde chese, for that is oftentymes the onely cause of the sayd stone. Al shelle fisshes are to be auoyded excepte it be a creuysshe, or a shrympe, measurably taken.

Ye muste, also take hede that ye eate

The regyment

no pepper nor hote spyces, nor no meates that are salte, sowre, or heuye of digestion, & that ye lye not on your backe on nyghtes when ye are a slepe. And ye oughte to kepe your reynes colde and moyst, & to let your backe be vntrussed in the somer.

After ye haue vsed this regiment or diete by a certayne seasō, it shalbe good for you to take an ounce of cassia newly drawen out of the cane, & eate it wyth a litle suger in the mornynge.

This ye muste vse euerye seconde weke, tyl in tyme your reynes be metelye wel clensed of the same, and euerye daye eate a lytle cassia, vpon a knyfes poynte, to kepe your bellie moyste: for that is one of the thinges that are most requyred in the sayd cure.

And at diuers other tymes when ye be disposed, ye maye take a litle of this receyte hereafter, whiche hathe greate vertue to mundifye the reynes, and to bringe the humours to equalitie, wyth releasing of the payne, and bryngynge
out

out the grauel.

⁋ A goodly sirupe to mundi=
fie the reynes.

Take the broth of a yonge chicken sodden tyl the bones fal a sondre thre pounde, melon seedes a litle bruſed, an ounce, percelye rootes, and aliſaundre rotes .iii. ounces, damaſke prunes, ſ: pe= ſten, of eche .vi. in nōbre, great rayſyns halfe an ounce, cleane licorice .x. dram= mes, waters of borage, endyue, and hop= pes, of eche .iii. drammes, and with suf= ficient white ſuger, boyle them al vnto the conſumption of the halfe and more, and afterwarde ſtreyne them, & make a goodly eſirup.

This is a thinge of excellent opera= tion, and an hye ſecrete in mundifyinge of the reynes, if ye kepe the diete as is afore described. The doſe of it is one cyath or a lytle cupful in the morninge earlye, and ſlepe after it a lytle. If ye wolde haue the forſayd ſirupe to purge more choler, then put in it a dramme of fyne reubarbe, with a lytle caſſia,

Hereafter

The Regyment

¶ Here after foloweth a pouder of excellent operation in breakynge of the stone.

Take the kernels that are within sloes, & drye them on a tyle stone, then make of them a pouder by it selfe, after that take the rotes of alisander, percelye, parietarie, and hollihocke, of euery one a like moch, and seeth them al in whyte wyne or els in ye broth of a yonge chycken, then streyne them out into a cleane vessell, and when ye drinke of it, adde as moche of the sayd pouder as ye thynke conuenyent, halfe a syluer spooncfull or more, for wythout dout it hath great effect in bryngyng out the grauell.

¶ An other expert medicyne for them that haue the stone.

There groweth in the galles of some oxen, a certayne yelowe stone, somtymes in bygnesse of a walnut, somwhat longe and bryttle. Yf ye take that stone and make of it a pouder, and eate it in your pottage, the weyght of one scrupule

pule or more accordyng to your strength it is a singuler medicyne to them that can not pisse for stopping of ye conduites

ℂ An other singuler medicine for the stone.

Take the seedes of smallache, perecelye louage, and sarifrage, the rootes of philipendula, chery stones, gromell seede, and brome seede, of euerye one a lyke moche, make them in fyne pouder, and whē ye be diseased with the stone, eate of this pouder a sponefull at ones in pottage, or in brothe of a chycken, and eate nothyng after .ii. or .iii. houres.

ℂ The xii. chapter, of remedyes for the goute.

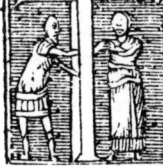

The payne in the ioyntes of a mans bodye, as in the handes and fete, is generally called arthritis, or gout, which procedeth somtyme of debylitie of ye synowes being lasshe and vnable, to consume the humours, that continuallye to

The Regyment

do flowe vnto them.

And for the moost parte they are all deryued from the member mandant, ẏ is to saye the brayne, for he is verye grosse, and engendreth euer humours in him felfe, by reason wherof, moche of the sayde humours are deriued into the nuke and muscles of the backe, and fro thence they descende into the feete, and then it is called podagra, or to the huckle boone, and then it is sciatica, or els into ẏ handes, ẏ there it is chiragra.

¶ Remedye.

For asmocheas all the sayd kyndes commeth of one begynnynge, as is shewed afore, and for the better expeditiõ in that we wyll be brefe, ye shall fyrste take awaye the superfluous moysture of the brayne, whyche is the roote and fountayne of all the sayd diseases, and that ye may do four emaner of wayes.

¶ The fyrst is obseruaunce of dyete inclynyng towarde drynesse, ẏ to auoyde all fulnesse of meate and drynke, and not to slepe in anye wyse shortlye after meate

of lyfe. fol. lxxix

meate. And ye must beware that ye eate no vaporous meates, nor thyn wyne, nor drynke moche after supper. And yf perchaunce the peyne be very sharpe, it shalbe moche holesome to the pacient, to abstayne from all kyndes of wyne, & to vse hym selfe to small drynke, which thynge yf he can not do, then let hym drynke claret wyne myxed with a good quantitye of water.

The seconde is to purge the brayne ones a moneth, wyth the one halfe of pylles of cochyes, and an other halfe of pylles assagareth. And in tyme of haruest, and of somer, with pilles sine quibus, and pilles imperiall, whereof ye shal gyue one dramme the nyght before the full moone, and the daye folowyng ye maye gyue hym to eate a lytle broth of cicers, with a lytle quantitie of raysyns of the sunne.

The thyrde is to represse the fumes, that ascende in to the brayne after meat which thyng maye well be done by easynge of a lyttle dredge, made of anys
seed

The regyment
seed and coriander.

The fourth is to parfume the brayne
with certayne thynges confortatyue,
as for example thus.

⁋ A good perfume agaynst moistures of the brayne.

Take fyne frankensence, sandrake
and mastike, of euery one an ounce, lignum aloes, a dramme, make them all
in grosse pouder, and parfume therewith stoupes made of flaxe or of cotten,
and laye vpon the head.

And when ye haue by this meanes
well, and dulye comforted the brayne, &
defended of, the originall cause of her
sayde disease, ye shall procede to take
awaye the matter conioynt that is descended vnto the synowes, and ye shall
begynne thus.

Fyrst ye must preserue the body from
engendryng of humours, in taking euery mornynge next your hert a conserue
made of ahornes, and of floures of rosemary, mengled with a lytle nutmygge
and mastike, and yf ye be of power, ye
may

may drynke a good draught of ypocras or other spyced drynke, after meate at dynner and at supper.

Secondaryly, ye shall vnderstande, that whosoeuer doth entende to be holpen of the goute, he must euery yere be purged two tymes, preparyng fyrst the matter to dygestion with syrupe of stichados, and duabus radicibus, with the one halfe of waters of sage, prymroses and margerym, in maner of a spyced iulep wt cinamom, taken .v. cōtinual mornynges .ii. houres afore ye eate any other meate. And after that, ye muste receyue a dramme of pylles called arthretikes, or hermodactiles, or of bothe togyther egall portions. Or take halfe an ounce of diacartami two houres after nyght, and of diaturbyth, of euerye one two drammes, with a lytle syrupe of hisop.

The reste of the sayde curation shall be accōplished wt the applyinge of dyuers locall remedies, whereof there be sondrye kyndes & sortes here declared.

ye

The regyment

Ye ought to rubbe the place that is fore with oyle of roses and a lytle vynegre, & after sprinkle vpon the same, fyne pouder of myrtylles. Another playster also as hereafter folowerh.

⁋A playster for the goute.

Take of the emplayster called mellilote, ii. ounces, populeō an ounce and a halfe, redde roses, mirtilles, and floures of camomyl, of euerye one a drame, make a playster and laye vpon the goutye ioynt.

⁋Another.

Take the iuyce of colewortes and of walworte, and with beane floure, and pouder of redde roses, and the floures of camomyl, make a playster and lay it to the sore.

⁋Another.

Take oyle of roses, crumes of bread, yolkes of egges, & cowes mylke, wyth a litle saffron, seeth them togyther a lytle as ye wolde make a pudding, afterwarde sprede them vpon cloutes & laye vpon the sore.

In

An other.

Make lye of the ashes of rosemary, or of oke, or of beane stalkes, and boyle in it, sauge, moleyne, prymrose, camomyll, and mellilote, and receyue ꝑ fume vpon the sore place, or wette cloutes in ꝑ sayde decoction, presse them and laye them vpon the payne.

Al the sayd remedies are very good to swage the payne of the goute, after the whych done, it is necessary to go about the comforting of ioyntes and sinowes, and to that intent ye maye applye the grese of pyes, oyle of camompl and of althea or holihocke, oyle of a fox oyle of earthwormes, oyle of prymroses, turbentyne, oyle of gromel brayde, wherwithall, or with one or two of thē ye may annoynt the sore place, and comfort both the synowes and the ioyntes marueylously. Also this oyntment that foloweth is singuler good for the same purpose.

Take fyue or syxe handfulles of walworte and seeth them well in wyne,

then

The regiment

them strayne them, and wyth a lyttle waxe, oyle of spike and aqua vite: make an oyntment wherewith ye muste anoynt the place mornyng and euenyng euery daye.

¶ An other oyntment
for the goute.

Take a fatte goose, and plucke her, and trymme her as yf she shulde be eaten, then stuffe the bellye within wyth two or thre yonge cattes, well chopped in small gobbettes, with an handful of baye salte, then sowe her vp agayne, & let her rost at a small fyre, and kepe the dryppyng for a precyous oyntment, agaynst all kyndes of goutes, and other diseases of the ioyntes.

¶ Medicines for the goute appropriate in all cases.

Take cowes donge, and seeth it in swete mylke, and laye a playster to the goute hote.

Also the yolkes of egges, womans mylke, lyneseede, and saffron all togyther

of lyfe.　　　　　fol. lxxxii

ther in a playster, swageth the diseases of the goute.

And yf ye be disposed to breake the skinne, and to let the humours issue (as by suche manye one is eased) ye shall make a lytle playster of blacke sope, and aqua vite, which wyl blyster it without any great payne.

Also very olde harde chese cutte and sodden in the broth of a gambon of bakon, and afterward stamped with a lytle of the broth, and made in maner of a playster, is a singuler remedy for diseases of the goute and was fyrst practised of Galene the prince of all phicitions,

❧ A prayer to God for helpe, agaynst the perturbations of the mynde.

Lorde my God, almyghtye father and ruler of my lyfe, my health, my strength, my redemer, and protectoure, sende vnto me the heauenlye beautes beames of thy holy spirite, to illumine the darkenesse of my synfull herte, and to guyde me to thy holye place. Shewe me the light of thyne aboundaūt mercy (O Lorde) that I may no lōger sleape in deedly synne. O only father of lyght which in very dede dost lyghten euery man that commeth into this worlde, for thy great mercyes sake it maye please the, to lyghten the eyes of myne herte, and to endue me wyth the spyryte of grace, that I maye loke vppon myne owne synne, the greate offences wherewith I haue offended the, and to know ȳ in my selfe there is no maner strēgth, for to wythstande the death, but onelye through the. And I beseche the o Lord, to couer these my carnall eyes, that they se no vanitie, & gyue me thy grace, that I fall not into concupiscence, to thende I may eschewe a leuyl thynges, and gyue my mynde holly to the obseruacion of thy cōmaundementes. Lord God I beseche the, that syn maye neyther raygne nor tary in me, and that I be not subiecte to myne owne fleshly

fleshly appetytes, but that I may expel out of my thoughtes all vnlawfull lustes, so that my soule and al my minde, maye be set holly vpon the Lorde God suffre not my soule to be oppressed, but receyue me into the protection of thy holy hand, and despise not me thy simple creature, whom thou hast redemed with the precyouse blood of thyne only sonne Iesu Christ. Thy mercy O Lord is aboue all that thou haste made, for thou doest differ the punyshmēt of the wycked, yf perchaunce they wolde amende at last, thou louest all that thou hast made, and hatest none but for their owne iniquities. And whē the wicked turne agayne to the, and crye vnto thy holye name wyth all theyr hertes by t by thy mercy is ready to receyue them, euen as I moost detestable synner come wyth hert cōtryte vnto thy mercy this daye: that I maye obtayne remissyon of my sinnes, To the I crye out of the very depth z botome of myne hert, go not awaye from me my maker z redemer, but heare the supplicatiō of my prayer

L.i.   For

For thou art myne onelye hope & myne
enheritaunce in the lande of lyuers. I
haue synned. I haue synned (O Lorde)
and heaped vp iniquitie euen agaynste
heauen, and afore the. But I know=
ledge myne offences, and desyre mercye
accordinge to thy goodnesse. Destroy
me not (O Lorde) amonge synners,
nor let me not descend into the lake of
death, that I vnworthy creature being
made worthy onely by the bounteous=
nesse of thy grace, may from henceforth
lyue in thy commaundementes, loue,
honoure, and prayse the. For all
heauenlye powers, angels, thro
nes, and dominations, laude
and prayse thy holy name
worlde without ende.
Amen.

℩ Thus endeth the
Regiment of
lyfe.

Here

The preface.

Here beginneth a goodly bryefe treatyse of the Pestylence, with the causes, signes, and cures of the same: compoſed, and newly recognised by Thomas Phayer studious in Philoſophie and Phiſicke, to the ayde, cōfort and vtilitie of the poore.

To the good reader a preface of the authour.

After that god almightye, father & creatoure of all thynges, had by hys vnſearchable proupdēce, ordeyned mankynde to eternal feliciti, and ioye at the beginning, he thought it not ynough to haue created him of nothynge, a bodye mooſte excellent, perfect & pure both in mēbres & ſēſes, aboue all other his creatures here in earth, but alſo of his ineſtimable goodneſſe endewed him with dyuers and ſondrye gyftes of grace, as wytte, vnderſtandyng, mynde and reaſon,

The preface.

in, wherby he myght not onelye (as nere as is possible) approche vnto hym in the knowledge of hys heauenly maiestye (as concernyng soule) but aswell ymagine, searche and fynde oute, by all maner wayes, aydes, comfortes and remedyes, wherby also the body myghte be saued and defended, agaynste all assaultes of any thyng that shulde anoye it: so bounteous and plentyfull are hys giftes implanted in our nature, that of all creatures we myghte haue bene the happyest. But after that synne had entred into the worlde, and by synne deathe (as saynt Paul sayth) our corrupte lyuynges haue made vs more corrupte, so that nowe the lyfe whych we leade here is not only not very pleasaunt vnto the mooste of men, and yf it be to some, yet it is incertayne, mutable, and short, but to many other it is excedyng greuous, sorowfull, and tedyous, subiect to diseases, infortunes, and calamities innumerable, which for the moost part done encrease dayly, euer the iust vengeaunce

of

The preface.

of God fallyng vpon vs for our greate abhominatiõs, and without doubt wil euer more endure, vnlesse we do repent, and lyue in hys commaundementes.

And to passe ouer all the hole swarmes of so manye, bothe olde and newe diseases, wherwyth the bodye of man (alas for our synnes) is contynuallye tourmented and vexed, to speake nothynge of these common and familier infirmities, as lepryes, agues, cankers, pockes, goutes, palsyes, dropsyes, reumes, phtysis, and other oute of nũbre, whych as yf they had cõspyred to fight agaynst Phisitiõs, can scantlye be appeased w[i]th anye cure of medicyne, what payne or punyshmẽt can ther be ymagined to put vs in remembraunce of oure owne wyckednesse, cause vs to detest our abhominable liuynges, & to call for mercye wyth lamentable hertes, more then this only plage & scurge of god commonlye called y[e] Pestilẽce. Is there any syknesse y[t] is halfe so violet, so furious and so horryble, as this syckuesse is?

L.iii. What

The preface.

What disease is there in the worlde, so venemous in infectynge, so full of payne in sufferynge, so hastye in devouryng, and so dificile in curynge, as the plage is? And yet are we now adayes, so stubburne and so frowarde, or els so drowned in the myre of fylthy and carnall appetytes, that we nothynge do regarde these open and manifest tokēs of our condemnation in the syght of God, but apply our hole studies to perseuer in our sinnes euer worse & worse, wherfore it is no maruaple though the sayde disease encreaseth, but rather to be feared, that almyghtye God wyll poure hys indignation vpon vs, with some other kynde of plage, more vyolent and terrible then the same is.

But to them that doo repente, and put theyr onelye truste in hym, who can do but wonder at his infinite benignitie, and goodnesse, that euen in the myddest of all the sayde afflictions, proudeth them of remedyes, lest they shulde dispayre: cureth and amendeth all their

greuous

The preface.

greuous sores, languours & diseases, he created medicine euen out of the earth, & of the wyse man it shal not be despysed. And surely amonges al other sycknesse is there none so daungerous, as is the forsaide plage for any man to cure, by the waye of medicine, for it turneth it self in so many maner of kindes, sykenesses & fashions, that they that are infected, are many tymes deed, afore it can be knowen, that they haue the same disease. Whych thinge although many noble & mooste excellent learned men, haue in tymes past worthely consydred, & therupon accordyng to theyr singuler knowledge & industryes gyuen to them of God, haue written vpon the causes, signes & cures of the sayde disease, so exactly, so learnedly, & with so great eloquence, & cunnyng, that there semeth nothynge either to be omitted, or possible to be added, to the perfecte curation of the same, & so it wolde be harde for a man of my slendre witte, to inuente the thyng that they haue not inuented, moche more in

vayne

The preface.

vayne shulde I go aboute to wryte the same thinges that they haue written alredye: Yet notwithstanding forasmoch as this disease when it ones beginneth enfecteth none so moche, as the comon people, among whom it is not gruē to al men, to vnderstande the forsard volumes, yf they had them present, moche lesse can they get theyr health by theyr owne ymaginacions or experimentes, specially, whē almost no phisition will vouchesafe to visite any suche infected of the comon sorte (so great is the dauger of this cruell syckenes) by reason wherof, the pacientes cast them selues often times into despeyr, and so many of ẏ pore people creatures of god, whiche by good medicines myghte well ynough recouer for lacke of such knowlege, are vtterly destroyed & cast away, to the great pitie of all christen hertes, contynuall ruyne of the comon weale, wyth diuerse other greuous & huge incomodities, as is dayly sene where the sayde dysease rayngneth.

I ther=

The preface.

I therfore at ye reuerence of almightye god, and for the loue yt I beare vnto myne euen chriſten, accordyng to the talent wherwith ye lord hath endewed me, vnder the correction of my frendes ye phiſicians, haue taken out of dyuers & ſondry volumes, of the moſt famouſe authours, that haue moſt exactly wryten of the ſayd diſeaſe, one peculyer certen and compendiouſe treatiſe, addyng therevnto ſuche holſome and ſynguler remedies, as I my ſelfe haue proued & knowe to be effectualle, in curynge of the ſame.

Deſyryng god almyghtye, the onely authour and reſtorer of al health, ſo to guyde the hertes of his ſupplyauntes, that the ſayde medicines maye take effecte in them accordynge to his gyftes, and as for my labour, I do nothing deſyre, but the loue and fauour of the gentle readers, whom I praye god continnually to encreaſe in all goodnes.

What

A treatyse of

What is mente or signified by this woorde pestilence.

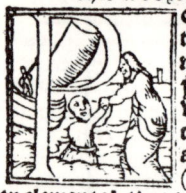

Pestylence is none other thyng but a venemous infectiō of ye ayer, enemye to ye vitall spirites, by a certayne maliciouse and euell propertye (& not of any qualitye clemental that is wythin it selfe.

For euen as pure triacle is a cōforter of lyfe not bicause of heat, cold, moystnes or drynes, but for as moch as oute of al his cōpositiō there redoūdeth a certayne fourme agreynge to the forme of the vital spirites of our body, so is the foresaid vapour enemy to our natures not for any qualitie as is sayde before, but for ye, ye his proporciō is directe euē cōtrarye to our vital spirites, cōsisting in ye harte, which vital spirites, yf by ye wil of God, & ordynary dyet, be strōger in the paciēt than ye forsayd vapour is they dryue it frō the bodye & wil not be infected,

the pestylence.

infected. And yf it happē that ẏ forsaid spirites be weaker thā the venym oꝛ the bodye ful of humours apte to putrefaction, than it doth incontinent assaute the lyuelye mēbꝛes, and excepte remedye, bꝛynge the body quycklye to destruction. But when we do saye the vapoure to be venemouse, we meane not that it is a poysō of it selfe in deede, foꝛ thē shulde euerye creature be indifferēt lye infected, ꝫ none shulde escape that dꝛaweth it in bꝛeath, but I cal it venymouse, foꝛ that it is of such a naughty qualitie that it may be lightlye conuerted into venyme, that is to say apte to burnynge and coꝛosion, as do mercury sublymed, quicke lyme oꝛ ratten bane, ꝫ other suche lyke kyndes of venyms.

¶Thus ye maye perceyue that all the great daunger ẏ is in this disease commeth of the noughtynesse of humours, which are made apte to receyue the said vapours, and not by violence of
the infected ayꝛe
nelye.

Of

A treatyse of
¶ Of the .iiii. rotes, or causes pricipal
of the sayde dissease, wherof it doth
arise & grow, & why it raygneth in one tyme, more
then in another.

The fyrste roote superior
and cause of the pesti-
lence is the wyll of god,
ryghtfully punyshynge
wycked men, of whyche
roote the holy scripture
treateth in manye places, as in Deu.
the .xxviii chapiter. If thou wylte here
the voyce of thy Lord God, and worke
and fulfyl all hys commaundementes,
the which I cōmaund to the this daye,
thy God shall make the more excellent
then all the people that be vpon the
earth. &c.

And in diuerse other places, he gyueth manye blessynges to thē that kepe
hys lawes.

And likewise to the people rebellyng
and breakyng hys commaundementes,
he

the pestilence

he thretneth many curses, as where he sayth.

If thou wylt not heare the voyce of thy Lorde God, to kepe and worke all hys commaundementes, whyche I cōmaunde the thys daye, there shall come vpon the these curses, and catche the. Thou shalte be cursed in the citye, and in the felde, thy barne shall be cursed, thy lyuynge shal be cursed, the frute of thy wombe shall be cursed, the frute of thy grounde shall be cursed, the heardes of thy shepe and thy cattel, shall be cursed, thou shalte be cursed at thy commynge in, and cursed at thy goynge out. Also a lytle after he sayeth. The Lorde shall ioyne to the the pestilence, til he hath c sumed the out of the erth. to the which thou shalt go to take possession. The Lorde shal stryke the with pouertie, feuers and colde, burnynge, and heate, and wyth a corrupt ayre. ʀc.

Also in an other place. The Lorde shall stryke the wyth the pestilence of Egypte, and the parte of thy bodye by
the

A treatise of
the whyche thou auoydeste thy donge, wyth a scabbe and ytche, and shalte not be able to be cured thereof, and let the heauen that is ouer the be as harde as brasse by cruell constellations, and the earthe on whyche thou doest treade, be lyke yron that euer wasteth, & waxeth worse and worse.

There be manye other maledictions whyche our Lorde hath threatned the rebellyous people wythall, expressed in manye places of holye scripture, but these may be sufficient as touching our entent, to shewe that manye tymes the cause of this disease is the vengeaunce of almyghtye God, ryghtfullye punyshynge men for theyr offences.

⁂ The seconde roote of the pestilence, whyche doth depende of the heauenlye constellactions.

Now

Nowe that we haue spoken of the fyrste rote superiour of the whyche thys dicease procedeth, it is also conuenient, that we declare somwhat of the seconde roote or cause superiour, that is to weete of naturall influences of the bodyes aboue.

And ye shall vnderstande, that accordyng to the sayinge of Marsilius ficinus (a man of excellente knowledge, & no lesse learnynge) in hys boke De triplici vita, & in an other whiche he wryteth also of the pestilence: that amonge al other heauenly bodyes, there be two bodyes called euyl and malicious, that is Saturne and Mars, whiche oftentymes by theyr vnholsome influences, are cause of manyfolde infirmytyes, specyallye of the pestilence. Saturne through colde, and Mars by excesse of heate. Saturne thorough colde, is the cause of reumes, of ye lepzye called elephācia, & al diseases commyng of colde matter,

Mars

A treatice of

Mars by reason of hys heate, bryngeth forth feuers pestilencial, spittyng of blood, water vnder the mydryfe, and the pleuresye, the whyche is a disease engendred lyke an aposteme of cholerycke matter in a thycke pannicle, or filme vnderneth the rybbes.

A prouident phisicion amonge many other thynges ought to cōsidre, the entring of the sūne into Aries, by true equacion of the houses and planetes, for that influence hath more domination, then haue al the other influences of the hole yere besyde, excepte the superiour coniunctions of the planetes, or els some greate eclyps. And thys entringe of the sunne into Aries, passeth al the entrynges of the sunne into anye other sygne.

Therfore you muste consydre howe the lorde of ♄. vi. house in the figure is disposed, for he is lorde of sychenesse, that is to say, you muste consydre whether he be impedyte or no, and yf he be impedyte, there shal be many sychenesses,

the pestilence.

ses, accordynge to hys nature and hys house, that is the .vi. house, as by exãple thus.

Be in case that Saturne is the lorde of the .vi. house, and some earthy sygne is in the same house, then mooste commonlye the sycknesse of that yere, shall be of lyke nature, that is colde & drye.

And ouer thys thou must consydre, whether that the lorde of the .vi. house hath any aspecte wyth the lorde of the house of death, or the lorde of the house of death to hym, then moost commonly the ende of those sycknesses that are colde and drye shalbe death.

And lykewyse as it is declared of the entrynge of the sunne into Aries, so it must be sayd of the coniunctions of the sunne and moone, thorough al the yere, markynge euer the nature of the planet beynge in the .vi. house, yf there be any, and the aspectes to those two houses aforesayd .&c.

Also he must consydre, whether thys entrynge of the sunne into Aries, or any

M.i.

A treatyse of

nye of the coniunctions of the luminaryes, be in the eyght house or no, for thē it shulde be moche worse.

And note, that yf the eclypse of the sunne or moone, be in any of the angles of the natiuitye of any person, or in any of the angles of the reuolucion of hys natiuitie, then he shal suffre sycknesse accordyng to the nature of the same angles. And yf the sayde eclypse be in the myddeste of heauen, he shall suffre hurte in hys honoure and fame, and yf it be in the ascendent, he shal be greued in hys bodye, and so forth of other houses, but it shalbe the worser, in case the eclypse be in the ascendent, specially yf it be the eclypse of the sunne, for ꝑ is the more daungerous of the two, for asmuch as ꝑ effecte of the eclipses of the mone, is alwayes fynyshed in the space of one yeare at the mooste, sometyme in lesse, and for the mooste parte in three monethes. But the effect of the eclipses of the sunne, is very longe or it come to passe, somtime, xii. yeres, as wytnesseth

Pto=

the pestilence.

Ptolome in hys centiloquio.

¶The Astrologians take the iudgement of the yere, by the entrynge of the sunne into Aries, in the fyrste minute, & yf it then happen that all the vl planetes be in the eyght house, whyche is the house of death, they saye that yere shall ryse a pestilence, and diuers other sicknesses, accordyng to the nature and condition of those planetes.

And yf the moone in the same entrynge be nere vnto the coniunction of ☉ sonne, as somtyme happeneth, within .ii. or thre or foure degrees, that yere shalbe a death and pestilence vniuersal, and that shortly after that coniunction specially at the commyng of the moone and the euyl planetes to infortunes, & as the infortunes be, the effectes shall so appeare, be they more or lesse.

Furthermore, ye muste consydre the great coniunction of the .ii. hyer planetes, as was ye coniunction of Saturn and Iupiter, the yere of our lorde. M ccccc.xxv, in the laste daye of August, &

M.ii. the

A treatise of
ye .xiii. degre of Scorpio: which coniunction chaunged from an ayrye triplicitie to a watry, & it was in a watrye sygne, whereof there chaunced verye moche rayne, & thervpon folowed the excessyue humectation or moystyng of mannes bodye, whyche by and by turned to putrefaction, and therevpon ensued peryllous & corrupte feuers, pestilences, and agues, specyallye bycause in the coniunction, Saturne was exalted, in the north aboue Jupiter, whyche Saturne is of yl influence.

¶ Of the thyrde roote or cause of thys outragious sykues.

The thirde rote or cause being inferiour, is the stynch and fylthye sauours that corrupte that ayre whyche we lyue in, for we can not lyue without drawynge of the breath, & we haue none other breth but of ye ayre rounde aboute vs whyche yf it be stynkynge, venymous and corrupte, and we
by

the pestilence,

by necessitie drawe the same vnto vs, immediatly corrupteth & enfecteth the harte, & the lyuely spirites of the same, and after y̅ iuuadeth al the other membres of the body to enfect them in likewyse, by reason wherof, is engendred a corrupte and venymous feuer of pestilence very contagious to all that are aboute them, for the venymous ayer it selfe, is not halfe so vehement to enfect as is the conuersation or breath of them that are enfected alreadye, and that by reason of the agreynge of the natures, whyche is the verye cause why our bodyes be infected by contagyon of men, more then any other beastes.

¶ Of the fourth roote or
cause of the sayd
disease.

The fourth rote is, the abuse of thinges not natural, that is to wete of meate and drynke, of slepe and watching, of labour and case, of fulnesse and emptynesse of the passions of the mynde, & of the immoderate

A treatyse of

moderate vse of lechery, for the excesse of al these thinges, be almoste the chefe occasion of all suche diseases as rayne among vs nowe a dayes.

For al that of our meate and drynke, is not dygested, turneth anon to putrefaction and to euyll qualities.

And to muche slepe replenysheth the body wyth to great aboundance of humours, but ouermoche watchyng doth drye vp the naturall humidities.

And as watchyng doth, so doth immoderate labour, and as slepe doth, so doeth rest and ease out of measure, put the bodye in greate distemper, and maketh it apte vnto this syknes, as is daylye sene.

And who so wil be ruled as becometh hym in thys case, shall neuer be lyghtly infected, and if chaūce be, he shall caselye wyth a lytle helpe, ye sometyme by verye nature onlye, saue him selfe and ouercome the syckenes.

Nowe seyng that the causes of this sayde disease be so great as is afore rehersed,

the pestilence.

hersed, it is not to be wōdered, though the thyng it selfe be verye huge & dangerous, and of harde curation, wherfore sayeth Auisen in hys fyrste of methaphisykes (although he were no christian) we muste wyth good and vertuouse lyuyng mitigate the wrath of god and by continual prayers kepe our selues styll in the state of grace.

Therefore wolde I councell euerye christen man, that is in dout of this disease, to cure fyrst the feuer pestilential of hys soule, callyng for þ holsome water þ wel of lyfe, wherof it is written.

Omnes sitientes venite ad aquas. &c. Whiche waters he onlye gyueth, that sayde to his disciples. Qui biberit ex aqua q̃ ego dabo illi:erunt i ventre eius a que viue salientes in vitam eternam.

And this done vndoubtedlye the sykenesse of the bodye shall be the easyer to be cured.

And for bycause the other soueraygne remedy preseruatyue is to flye the corrupte ayre, accordyng to the prouerbe,

M.iiii. Longe,

A treatyse of

Longe, cito tarde. Flye be tymes, flye farre, and come slowelye agayne.

¶ Yet for so muche as euerye man can not, nor is of abilitye so for to do, it is good for them to loke vpon thys lytle regiment, wherin wyth the ayde of almyghtye god the hye Phisition, yf the venyme be not to outragyouse, he shall fynde howe to preserue hym selfe well ynough from it.

And for the better knowlege and vnderstandynge of thys treatyse, ye shall knowe þ it is deuided into .ii. partes.

¶ The first is of the maner to preserue a manne from the pestilence only by dyet, in suche thynges wythout the whyche, one can not be longe alyue in healthe

¶ The seconde treateth of the cure of the sayd disease by the waye of holsome medycine.

¶ The fyrst parte is distribute into .vii. lytle chapters.

¶ The fyrste chapter treateth of the election of the ayer.

Th

the pestilence

⁌ The.ii.of meates and drinkes.
⁌ The.iii.treateth of sleapynge and of wakynge.
⁌ The fourth treateth of excercyse
⁌ The fyfth of emptynes and fulnes.
⁌ The syxte speketh of the accidentes of the mynde.
⁌ The.vii. of medicines preparatyue.

 The seconde parte is deuy=
  ded in to.vi.chapters.

⁌ The fyrste howe to knowe whan a man is infected.
⁌ The seconde of the cure of the pesti= lence by the waye of dyete.
⁌ The thyrde of the cure of the pesty= lence by the power of medicines.
⁌ The.iiii.of cure thereof by lettynge of blood, ventoses, and purgations.
⁌ The.v.of the cure of the same by out warde applications.
⁌ The.vi.howe to cure the botche cal- led a Carbuncle, or Anthrax.

 ⁌ The fyrst chapter of the fyrst
  parte, treating of the elec=
   tion of the ayer.

       Although

A treatyse of

Lthough the disposition of the ayer cold and drye, or els moderately moiste, be moche comendable in the tyme of pestylence, yet there muste be moderatiō in the same, as well as in the .vi. thynges not natural heretofore declared. For ye muste haue a good respecte vnto the complexion, the age, the custome of lyuinge, þ region, cōpositiō of þ bodye, strēgthe, syckens tyme, and many other thynges.

For some requyre an ayer more hote, than other some do, and lykewyse in other thynges, the whyche I do remyt vnto the good discretion of euerye wel lerned man, and to suche other as haue any knowlege of naturall thynges.

For the more suerty it is good for them þ may, to dwell in hygh or hylly groundes, hauyng in the mornyng whan the sunne is vp, a wyndowe open towarde

the

the pestilence

þ cast, & whan the sonne goeth downe, an other wydowe open to ward þ west and close vp all the wyndowes on the south syde, for that wynde is verye yll in tyme of pestilence.

Also it is good to rectifye the ayre wythin the house, yf it be in somer, by spryncklynge in the chamber vyneger, & water of roses, if it be wynter or colde make a lusty fyer of clene wood, & put in it encence, myrre, laurel tre, or iuniper, or cypres, and in tyme temperate, myngle the hote thynges wyth þ colde aforesayde

Whyche sprincklynges, and burnynges, ye maye make at all tymes whan ye wyll, but specially in the mornynge, to correcte the vapoures of the nyghte.

I rede in Plotyne, that the egiptians were wonte to fume their houses and theyr bodyes in the daye wyth turpentiue or rosin and in the nyght with mirre caste vpon the coales and so resisted al venymous ayres & contagions.

The fyrste hathe so greate vertue a-
gayn

A treatyse of

gaynst the pestilence, that we rede how Hypocrates preserued the hole coūtrye and citye of Athenes, by makynge of greate fyres in the stretes, and al about the towne by nyght, and so delyuered them from the certayne death ý shulde haue comen amonge them. For whyche cause the citizens of the sayde towne, made vnto hym an ymage all of golde, and honoured hym alyue as yf he had bene a god.

And it is good in hote time, to strowe the chambre ful of wyllowe leaues, and other fresh boughes, which must be gathered after the sunne settyng, & lay about your bedde & windowes, vine leaues, quinces, pomegranades, orenges, lymons, citrons, and such other frutes, that are odoriferous, as roses, floures, of nenuphar, violettes, and other lyke.

And in colde tymes, take sage, laurell, minte, wormewood, nept, bawme, rue, and galingale, whyche thynges ye maye sometyme cary aboute wyth you in a cloth to take the ayer of them.

And

the pestilence.

And in tyme of heate, temper a sponge or a cloute in water of roses, and vynegre. And in tyme of colde ye maye adde to it a lytle cinamome, and thus he that is disposed to haue precioufe sauours, as pomeaunders, or other such may compose them accordynge to necessytie, & as the complextō of hys body shal requyre.

Alway takyng hede the women whiche are with chylde, and they that haue the suffocation of the mother or els catarres, take no such odour, as shal put theselues to any daunger, or displeasure.

In a colde tyme it is good to holde in the mouth, zedoary, enulacampana, cynameme, cloues, the rynde of a citron lignum aloes, or any one of them. But yf the season of the yere be hoote, then take corianders prepared, graynes of paradyse, saunders, seedes of orenges, or of lymons. And in temperate wether, myngle the one with the other.   But it is good in all tymes, to bere aboute you precioufe stones, (yf ye haue them) speciallye a iacincte, a rubye, a garnet,
an

A treatyse of

an emeralde, or a saphyre, whyche hath a speciall vertue, agaynst the pestilence, and they be the stronger, yf they be borne vpon your naked skynne chyeflye vppon the fourth finger of the left hand for that hath greate affinitie wyth the hart aboue other membres.

And as touchynge them that are cōtynually amonge the sycke of thys disease, they must take hede in any wyse, to kepe them from theyr breathe, and that they do not stande betwene them and the fyer, nor receyue the odoure of theyr swettes, vrynes, vomites, and other excrementes of the bodye nor to eate and drynke with them, nor in their vessellcs, nor to lye in theyr couches, nor weare any of theyr apparell, except they be well psonned, or wethered in ye cleane ayer.

It is also good to flye from all places that be corrupte, or stynkynge, and to kepe the stretes & houses very swete and cleane. And the rulers ought so to prouyde, that no filthy donge, nor anye deade

the pestilence.

deade caryons, be caste into the stretes, for that shulde sore enfecte the ayer, & brynge many men to death. And during al the time of thys disease, there ought to be no hote houses vsed, but forbiddē and locked vp, tyl such tyme they se no further daunger.

¶ The seconde Chapter, of eatyng and drynkyng

He meates oughte to be of very lyght digestiō, more i somer thē i wynter, hauing alwaye an eye vnto the cōplexions, customes and other thynges aforsayde.

¶ The houre what tyme ye shal receyue your meate, is when your appetyte cūmeth vpon you, after the fyrst digestiō made. Greate repletion ought to be abhorred, but a sufficient meale is verye holsome. Neither is diuersitie of meates alowed of anye physike, but yf ye wyll haue diuers sortes, then begynne wyth

A treatyse of

wyth them that are the lyghtest to dygest, and that best nourisheth the body.

Your breade muste be of pure corne kepte in good ayer, and not fusty, metely well salted, wyth sufficient leuen, & baken in a place where none euyll ayer is, and it must be of a daye or two dayes olde, or there about,

Wheate is beste amonge al other cornes, euen as wyne amonge all other licours, although the barlye breade be good for thē þ minde to kepe thē leane.

Meates of euyll taste, after they be longe dead, and stynkyng fyshe in lyke maner, and the fattes of all fyshes, and meates þ haue ben twise sodden, thicke wyne and troublous, or otherwyse corrupte, waters of marishes, and blacke groundes, and al such corrupte meates and drynkes, be very peryllous.

But good wyne, sauoury, and cleare and good meates taken wyth an appetyte are cause of health, and preseruation from the pestilence.

Vinegre is a noble thyng in tyme or pestilence,

the pestilence.

tion from the pestilence.

Vinegre is a noble thyng in tyme of pestilence, yf ye haue none other impedimēt to let you to receyue it, & ye may correct it, accordynge to the nature of ye cause, in suche wyse, as may be comfortable to the vital spirites of the harte.

Borage and buglosse, are very good preseruatyues in this case, and so is a lytle quantitie of saffron, orenges, lymbs, pomgranades, citrons, prunes of damaske, and other suche, in good conuenient quantitie, addynge to them a lytle suger, and cynamome for correction.

A nutte is called the triacle of ruthe, shaled & sugered wyth a lytle rose water, and as sayth Isaac, a nut & a fygge drye taken afore dynner, preserueth a man from al maner of poysons.

⁋ The thyrde Chapter, of slepynge and watchyng.

N.i.   To

A treatyse of

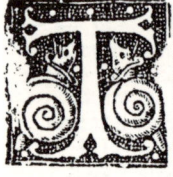

TO moche slepe engendreth many humours in ye body, specially if it be i the day tyme, & it dulleth ye memory, and maketh a mā vnlusty & apte to receiue ye pestilēce. Therfore created almyghtye God ye nyght, wherin we shulde rest,& the day for to kepe vs wakyng ye we fal not ito synne and slouth. Surely to slepe on ye daye tyme is exceadyng hurtfull, for whē the sūne ryseth, he openeth the poores of the body, and bryngeth the humours and spirites from within, to the outward partyes, whyche prouoketh a man to watchynge, and exceercyse or workes.

And contrary wise when the sunne goeth downe, al thynges are closed and coacted, whyche naturally prouoketh a man to reste.

Moreouer, the stomake by the vehement heat of the day is naturally dilated and spredde abrode, so euer agaynst nyght,

the pestylence.

nyght, by reason of the auoydasice of þe spirites it waxeth somewhat feble, and when the nyght commeth, requireth to haue quyete, whereby it maye acquyre more plentye of spirites for the nouryshynge of it selfe.

And therfore whosoeuer waketh in the tyme of slepe, or slepe whē he ought to wake, he peruerteth, and hurteth not onely hys memorye, & al hys other vertues of the mynde, but also manye tymes shal engendre apostemes, catarres, reumes, agues, palsyes, & many other greuous & naughty diseases in þe body.

Also ye must take hede, þ ye watche not to muche, for thereof cūmeth dryneffe of the brayne, & many other sykenesses, that melancholye bredeth. But he that is vsed to slepe very moche, and can not abstayne in anye wyse, let hym slepe in a chayre, or elles syttynge in a place that is colde, but not lyinge, yf he loue his health.

¶ The Fourth Chapter,
of exercyse.

A ii.   No

A treatise of

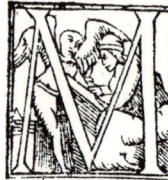

Moderate exercyse or laboure is verye necessarye to the preseruynge of healthe, accordyng to every mānes age, custome, cōplexiō, strēgth & such other, so it be done ī the mornynge, and at euen, before anye meate, and in a place of good ayer, and not infected with corruption.

Auicenne sayth, that he onely ought to abstayne from laboure, that nothyng regardeth the health of his bodye.

And Galene sayeth ÿ exercyse quycketh ÿ vertues natural, animal, & vital.

And Rasis telleth of a great pestilence, wherin there were very fewe saued, bicause they liued ydely, and wold do no labour.

Finally defaute of good exercise is oftentymes the cause that manye dye sodely, afore they fele thēselues sick, &c.

⁂ The .v. Chapter of emptynesse and fulnesse.

It

the pestilence.

It is holesome for you, euery daye once to procure ẏ ducty of the wōbe yf ye can not naturally, yet at ẏ leste wayes seke some other meanes, as by a glistero, suppositorye, for the lōge wythholdynge of anye superfluytyes, is in this tyme very daungerous & hurtfull. And all the tyme the sayde disease endureth, they that haue any fistules, ought not to be cured.

And they that haue anye yssues by their hemoroides, maye not be restrayned without the fluxe be sore excessyue, & they that had the forsaid hemoroides and were cured afore, let them open thē agayne, for feare of further daunger.

Also they ẏ are disposed to be scabbye, hauyng great ytche, and suche diseases of the skynne, ought to bryng the matter out by rubbynge, and vehement clawynge wyth theyr nayles.

Excesse of women, is exceadynge peryllous, but yf ye can not rule your
N.iii.   selfe,

A treatyse of

selfe, take good hede, ye do nothynge a=
fore the fyrste digestion, and tyll nature
doeth prouoke you, for euerye suche ex=
cesse weakeneth more the body, then yf
ye shulde be let blood. xl. tymes so much
as wytnesseth Auicenna, & is cause ma=
ny tymes of pestilence, and of death.

¶ The. vi. Chapter, of acci=
dentes of the mynde.

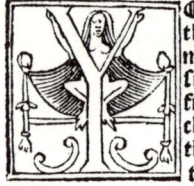

WE must beware of al
thynges that shulde
make you to be pen=
sife, heauye, thought
full, angrye or melan
cholycke, for all such
thynges are ynough
to enfecte a man a=
lone.

Passe the tyme ioyfullye in good thin
ges honest and decent, euerye mā accor=
dynge to his owne herte, and the estate
that God hath called hym vnto.

¶ The. vii. Chapter, of medi=
cynes preseruatyues.

the pestilence.

ALL they ꝑ are of good cõplexion and of holsome diete, nede not to be purged. For an hole body and voyde of all humours, is not lyghtlye taken of the pestilence, as the other are.

But yf it be a bodye full of humoures, or a great eater without any exercyse or trauayle, such ought to let them selues be purged, and they that haue to moche quantitie of blood, or yf ꝑ blood be any thynge corrupte, they ought to aske counsayl of some good expert phisicions, and not to put theyr trust in any vayne bosters that detracte other, whyche in all cases and at all tymes, gyue them mercury precipitant, and other medicines corrosiue, which for the moost parte are venyme of them selues and vnder colour of an other medicyne do disceyue the pacient, a wonder to beholde, how craftely they couer it, some tyme in syrupe, sometymes in sugre, or

A.iiii.   ther-

A treatyse of

therwhyles in fygges, lozenges, or ra=
syns, leste it shoulde appeare (as it is in
dede) that they gyue the pacientes very
quyck syluer. Some other affirme that
the mercurye is quenched, or throughly
mortifyed, & worketh none other wyse
but by secrete qualitie agaynst all dis=
eases in the bodye of man, for the ex=
cesse of elementes saye they, is clerelye
corrected in prceipitacion and adustion
of the fyre. How commeth it to passe (if
this be true) that when a lytle of it is
set vpon a cole and a pece of fyne golde
adioyned to it, we may se playnely the
very quyckesyluer, cleuyng to the gold
and wyll make it as brittle as yf it had
lyen in very rawe mercurye? Yea howe
chaunceth it that when it is mengled
w hote creame, it wyll be crude agayne
as it was afore. And to saye the truthe
the quycke syluer rawe, is better to be
dronken, then suche as is sublimed, for
that hath ben permytted, both of dios=
corides and of dyuers other: But we
neuer red of any good phisicion that e=
uer

the pestilence.

uer gaue counsel to take the precipitate bycause of the copporose and other venymous ingredience being with it.

And although that for the tyme peraduenture some escape, & fele not theyr effect in dede as many other do (that is to saye, debilite of the vertue radicall of the stomacke and other mēbres principall, purgyng of the good humours & leauynge the euyll within the bodye, wherof ensueth tmanytymes death) yet they leaue a certayne euyll qualitie or impression of the bodyes in all that do receyue them, and so they make worke for good phisicions, to the greate hurte of them that haue beleued them.

Suche galautes shulde go proue theyr pouder made of quycke syluer, amonge the Turkes and Sarysins, & not vpon theyr euen chrysten, and theyr neyghbours. But now to our entent.

The pylles called pillule cōmunes, aboue other pylles preseruatyues, are alowed to be of hyest operation, by reason of a certayne propertye that they
haue

A treatyse of

haue within them, as Rufus the composer of them sayth, that he neuer saw anye man that vsed them, but he was preserued from the pestilence.

¶ There goeth into theyr composition myrre and aloes, which haue great vertue to kepe the body from putrefaction and are made thus,

¶ Take of aloes epatik wel washed.ii drammes, myrre walshed, and saffron, of eche a dramme, make them vp wyth whyte wyne, or the iuyce of lymons, or of orenges and sugre.

Some take them euery thyrd day, the weyght of halfe a dramme, in the mornyng.iii.pylles, and euerye daye one afore supper. Let euery man do accordig to his nede, and as his bodye is replete with humours, but it is good to drinke after them a good draught of wyne, tempered in a lyttle water of roses, or of wormewoode, and yf they be to harde, let them be resolued in the sirupe of lymons, or a lytle wyne.

Some doctours ioyne vnto them other

the pestilence.

ther spyces, after the cōplexion of the person, and the humour that they nede to purge. And they wash the aloes and the myrre, in an hote season, & for hym that hath an hote lyuer, in water of roses & of endiue, but in that let euery mā be his owne iudge, yet I wolde counsell them to stycke rather to the good experimentes þ haue ben accustomed, thā þ fantesies of their owne ymaginaciōs

The Apoticaryes ought to haue in store both the two sortes, and to se that they be sufficiently leuened, and that þ foresayde aloes be clect and pure.

They whiche haue the hemoroydes & wolde vse the foresayd pilles, let them adde a lytle mastyke, or the gūme that is called bdellium. Yf any haue a bloodye fluxe, or excoriation of the bowels, let him not receyue them without a better counsell. Women also greate with chylde, and they that are subiect to any fluxe of blood, ought not to receyue thē

Amonge other thynges it is a good preseruatiue, and a thynge well expert
and

A treatyse of

and commended, to eate in the morning
fastynge one drye fygge, one walnutte,
and four or fyue leaues of rue, chopped
all togyther, and afterward to drynke
a draught of good wyne. But it shal be
sufficient for them that are with chyld
to take ye said thiges, leuing out ye rue.

In an hote season, it is good to temper the sayd wine with a lytle rosewater or of vyolettes. Some other take. v
houres afore dyner, thre tymes a weke,
the weyght of halfe a crowne of mithri
datū, or of fyne triacle, tempered in a litle good wyne. But in tyme of heate,
for hote complexions, it is good to put
in it a lytle conserua roses, and to men
gle them with water of sorell, or of borage, or of buglosse.

Mithridatum is a greate medicine agaynste all kynde of venymine, for we
reade that the founder of it, kyng Mithridates, who dyd vse to eate thereof
could neuer be hurt by any kind of poy
son. The same Mithridates beinge ouercome in battayle of the Romaynes,
wolde

the pestilence.

wolde haue kylled hym selfe wyth the mooste swyftest poyson that coulde be deuysed, but whē he had drōken many sortes of suche, & neuer a one wrought any thynge to purpose, he caused hym selfe to be slayne of his seruautes, after whose death Pompeius, the graūd capitayne of the hooste, founde in hys secret coffers, a certayne byll wrytten of his owne hande, in effects thus.

Twentye leaues of rue, two fatte fygges, two walnuttes, and a lytle salte, whosoeuer eateth of thys shall be sure from all kynge of venyme that daye.

The good triacle also hath a greate vertue, but there ought to be a punyshmēt of them that do abuse it with coūterfayted stuffe, which deceyue th many people, and causeth them to dye, that put theyr trust in it.

Some other take in tyme of colde, a cloue or ii. of garlyke, whiche is called the husbandmans triacle, & after drink a draughte of good wyne, and in hote tyme take and eate a fewe leaues of sorell,

A treatyse of

rell, and drynke a draught of the water thereof distilled, for it is excellent & good in all complexions, tymes & ages. Also it is good to drynke euerye mornynge a draught agaynst the pestilence that is thus made.

℟ A drynke for the pestilence.

Take in the moneth of June or at any other conuenient tyme, our lady thystle burnet, scabious, gentiane, sorel, of euery one a lyke moche, floures of buglosse redde roses, herbe dragons, and matfelon or morsus diaboli, twyse as moche as all the other, stepe them all in whyte wyne & rosewater, durynge one nyght, then set them all in a cōmon styllatory, wayinge in for euery pounde of herbes, halfe an ounce of bole armenic poudred augmētyng the proportion, accordyng to the quantitie of the herbes, then styl a water, and for euery pynt of it, take ye weyght of a crowne of saffron, halfe an ounce of yelowe saunders fynely poudred, and put them all in a violle wyth the foresayde water stopped, and sette them

the pestilence.

them in the sunne one moneth. This is a noble water for a mā whyche hath the pestilence, to drynke.

And he that wyll, may put a lytle sugre, and poudre of cinamome in it, that it may be more pleasaunt in the taste. He that can not fynde the sayde herbe called matfelon, or morsus diaboli in latine, let hym take ẏ double weyght of dragons. It hath a roote as it were halfe eaten of by the myddes, and it is so called, bycause the fable is, the deupl bytit of, for thenuy he hath to man, lest we shoulde obtayne the greate vertues of the same.

The horne of an vnicorne put in the drynke, bole or in pouder, hath a great effecte agaynst the sayde disease, and agaynste all kyndes of poyson.

¶ Here foloweth a very good preseruatyue for the cōmon
people, redye at all ty=
mes & of small coste.

Take an ounce of leaues of rue, halfan ounce of good fygges, one ounce of
Jenuper

A treatyse of
Juniper buries, two ounces of walnuttes pyked, iiii. ounces of vynegre, and a good quātitie of saffron, stampe all the foresayd thinges togyther, and reserue thē in an earthen cuppe, or a glasse faste stopped, that no ayre yssue, whereof yf ye receyue in the mornyng vpon a knyfes poynt, the quantitye of a beane, or more, ye shalbe sure by the grace of god not to be enfected in foure and twenty houres after.

⁋ An other pouder for the same.

Take pure and electe bole armonyacke, not counterfayte, but suche as is wythout grauel, smoth, somewhat shinynge, and to the eye a farre of mooste lyke a verye stone, not to bryttle, nor to hye coloured for such is commonly sophisticate. Take I saye the sayd bole armoniak, and grynde it vnto fine pouder, than wasshe it in whyte wyne or in rosewater, or water of buglos, sorel, or wormewood, or scabiouse, afterwarde drye it and pouder it agayne, and do so

b.oj.

the pestilence,

v.oz.vi.tymes, euer walſhyng, dzyenge and poudcrynge the ſame, and at laſte ſet it vp in a cleane veſſell, tyll ye nede to vſe it.

Men of hote complexion, yf they wil receyue it, muſte take of it a ſponefulle wyth vynegre, oz water of ſozell.

And they that be of colde complexion, maye take it in a lytle wyne, oz ſeabyouſe water in the moznynge. For it pzeſerueth the bodye, from all cozruption, conſumeth the ſuperfluouſe humours, and dzyueth awaye the venym from the herte.

¶ An other ſynguler remedye
pzeſeruatyue for ryche
men and delicate
of cōplexion.

Take zedoarye, lignum aloes, agrimonie, ſaffrō, ariſtologia rotunda, yf it may be gotté, whit diptany, gentian, the rinde of a citron, the ſeede of citron, of euerye one a ſcruple, cozianders pzeparat, turmentyl, red ſaunders, red coral, red roſes,

D i.   yuozye,

A treatyse of

ynowe, mirabolanes emblyke, of euery one a dramme, terra sigillata, two drammes, bole armonyake. iii. drammes, pouder al these, and wyth fine suger, & syrupe of acetositate citri, make a noble electuarye, and kepe it as a treasure of mannes health, in the tyme of pestylence.

⁋ An other souerayne & goodlye receyte bothe preseruatyue & curatyue.

Take a hennes egge, newely layde, and make an hole in the crowne, by þ whyche ye shall drawe oute all the whyte thereof, and leaue the yolke within the shell, which done fyll the same egge, wyth good englysh saffron hole, as moche as maye be stuffed in the shelle, than drye this egge agaynst the fier, or in an ouen, whan the bread is out, so longe tyll the shelle be vtterlye blacke and brent, and the reste sufficiently bryttle and drye, make it in pouder in a morter, and adde to it as muche

the pestylence.

muche pouder of mustarde sede as shal waye all the hole egge, than take thys ingrediens at the apothecaryes, Dytamy, turmentille, nux vomica, of eche a drāmme, pouder euerye one of them by it selfe, then put them altogyther, and put to it rewe, pionye roote, zedoarye, camphere, & fyne triacle of eche equall portion, so that the weyght of them .v. be asmoche as all the reste, beate them in a mortar by the space of .ii. houres, tyll all be incorporated togyther in a lumpe, than put it in a glasse, and kepe it, couered with a lefe of gold, in a cold place, for it wyll laste thus .xxx. yeres, without corruption, and is a thinge of inestimable value in this case, the dose of it to preserue, is but one halfepenye weyghte, or lesse, ye the weyght of one barlye corne, hath in it a marueylouse strength, in defendynge the bodye.

But yf one were infected aledy, than he muste receyue, afore lettynge blood ii. or .iii. graynes, after hys bleedynge, gyue hym in the name of god, an hole scruple,

A treatyse of

scruple, o?, ii. o?, iii. (yf hys strengthe wyll serue) tempered wyth wyne for a hote takynge, and in great colde wyth a litle aqua vite, and thervpon sweate.

❡ I haue knowen whan the syke hath bene vtterlye desperate, and coulde reteyne nothyng, yet by the grace of god, thorough the meanes of two scrupules hereof, myxte wyth a litle aqua vite, bothe the vomyte immedyatly ceassed, and nature recouered, escaped the daunger of death.

As concernyng swete waters to spryncle vpon your clothes and thynges of pleasaunte odoure, to be caste vpon the coles when ye aryse on mornynges, and also the makynge of good and holsom pomaunders, to smell vpon in tyme of pestilence, for the contentation of them that are desyrous, I shal here rehearse i. or. ii. of euerye sorte, to the entent ye maye (whan ye be disposed) eyther vse them, or deuyse other of the same makynge: as it shalbe requisite accordyng

to

the pestilence.

to necessitye.

¶ Fyrste a swete water that is made thus.

The water of roses: violettes or nenuphar, or one of them or of al togyther one pounde, good vinegre two ounces, maluesey, muscadyne, or other pleasaunte wyne, thre ounces, of bothe the saunders, of eche one dramme and an halfe, camphore, one scruple, and yf ye haue anye gallia muscata, adde thereto halfe a dramme, myngle them togyther, and spryncle vpon your clothes, when ye be disposed.

¶ The ryghte excellente, and famouse doctoure Iohannes Manardus also, in the thyrde epistle of hys fyfth boke, doeth shewe, howe to make in tyme of Pestilence, two soueraygne perfumes, the one for to seru: in sommer whyche is made thus.

¶ A Fumigation for somer.

D.iiii. Take

A treatyse of

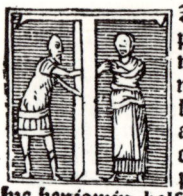

Ake redde ambre .ii. partes, the leaues of myrte, floures of nenuphar, roses, vyolets, saffron, maces, and yelowe sauders of eyther of them .i. parte, camphore, ambre, beniamin, halfe a parte, muske the tenth of one parte, myngle all togyther this is a pleasaunt and comfortable sauour in the tyme of somer.

But in winter season ye maye vse this.

Take storax calamita, yreos, mastyke, of eche two partes, cloues, maces, nutmygges, cynamome, saffron, of eche one parte, aumbre the fyfthe of one parte, muske the tenthe of one parte, myngle al togither and make a fumigation.

And of these pouders ye maye make lytle balles, or pomaunders, to beare aboute with you at al tymes, but the last receypte muste be wel incorporate wyth

a

the pestilence.

a lytle storax liquida, and lapdanum, & the other wyth lapdanum, gumme, dragagant, and rosewater.

¶ An other goodly pomaunder for gentlewemen and ladyes.

Take the rynde of an orenge, cloues, lignum aloes, of eche, one dramme, calamus aromaticus, halfe a dramme, alipta muscata one dramme, roses, myrtylles, of euery one halfe a dramme, nutmygge, cinamome, beniamin, of euery one a scruple make it vp in a morter, wyth Storax liquida, with sufficient waxe, and maluesey addinge in the ende, of camphore, halfe a scrupule or more.

And in the tyme of pestylence, ye ought to kepe the house euery daye til the sonne be vp, and yf it chaunce that ye go among a great multitude of people, where is a nye daunger to be feared: ye may chew a litle zedoarye in your mouth, ones in an houre or two, but holde it not conty

nuallye

A treatyse of

nuallye for hurtynge of the gummes.

zedoarie (as sayeth Auicenne in hys boke de viribus cordis) comforteth the harte, and engendreth good blood, it is holsome for the stomake (as affyrmeth Plinie) maketh good digestion, & prouoketh appetyte.

¶ Constantyne in hys booke of degrees, sayeth, it hath a great power agaynste venyme, and the stynkynge of the mouthe, it breaketh wynde, and cureth the bytinges of venemous beastes and serpentes.

When the sonne shineth in a cleare daye, ye maye walke in gardeynes medowes, hylles & by ryuers, but beware of lakes, standyng pooles, and fennes, for oftentymes the enfection of the ayre, aryseth of ye corrupte vapours, boylynge out of suche vnholsome places.

¶ The seconde parte, of the cure of one that is enfected with ye pestilence alreadye.

Howe

the pestilence

¶ Howe to knowe a mane that is infected, the fyrste chapter.

WE sayde i the beginning, how ẏ pestilence was engendred of ẏ corrupt and noughtie ayer, turning al the humours of the bodye quyckkye to corruption & to venyme.

Wherfore we muste take hede betymes, lest the vital membres be infected of the sayd poyson, for it euer seketh to the herte, and yf it come vnto the herte, afore the medicyne, then is there no recouery, for not one amonge an hundred lyueth. For the sayde venyme is so swyfte, so fearce, and so boystous of it selfe, that it wyll not (withoute greate difficultie) be put out of possession, but dryueth awaye the medicyne from the herte agayne.

But yf the medicyne come vnto the hert afore the venyme hath the vpperhande, then he dryueth it oute, by the helpe

A treatyse of

helpe of the vertue expulsyue, of the spyrituall membres, and that expulsiō commonly is by swette.

And forbycause somtimes a man is poysoned, ɫ can not tel hym selfe, nor none that is about him, wherof manye daūgers doth arise, for as the prouerbe is, one scabbye shepe enfecteth a hole flocke, therfore it shal be necessary that euerye man take hede vnto hym selfe, ɫ consydre al the sygnes and tokens that shal be sayd hereafter, for the more care that he hath about that, the soner shall he escape out of the daunger.
And yf a man feleth hym selfe enfecte, aboue al thyng let hym remembre god, for it is a sycknesse that in a twynklinge of an eye may brynge a man to death.

Fyrst let hym loke, whether in hys arme holes, flankes, or vnder his necke there be any aposteme or swellynge, or whether in any other partes of hys body there appeare anye grene, blacke, or euill coloured sore, for that is the signe that neuer fayleth, but the person certaynly

taynly is enfected. Notwythstandyng
every man enfected with the pestilence
hath no suche vlcers, botches or sores,
wherfore ye muste take hede of ẏ other
signes hereafter, that ye be not deceyued for lacke of the sayd apostemes.

But what is the cause that suche apostemes somtymes doth appeare, & somtymes doth not: no doubt, but bycause
that when the venym is so vehement &
so furious, and hath gotten hold in the
bodye of man, nature by reason of the
swyftenesse of the infection, is so troubled, letted, and entangled, that she cannot tell which waye to succour, and so
can dryue out none apostemes, & that is
more perillous, then yf there were many sores. But agayne, when the venym
is but meanely furious, & the nature of
ẏ pacient strong ynough by reason of
good humours, then it defendeth it self
and dryueth the venym from the hert &
principall membres, to suche places as
it maye be best auoyded at, which breaketh forthe by compulsion in botches,
carbuncles

A treatise of
carbuncles and other sores.

¶ The seconde sygne, is, yf ye feele a greate pryckynge and shotynge in your bodye, and specyallye in any of the .iii. clensyng places, that is to say the neck, the armeholes and the flankes.

¶ The thyrde sygne is when ye fele an outragyous heate within you, as yf ye were in the fire. Which heate somtyme spreadeth it self abrode through al the hole bodye, and otherwhyle there aryseth suche a colde, that it maketh a man to shake as yf he were in a feuer. Wherin al ye that be infected must take hede: for some there be that in the begynning fele not such a feruent heate outwardly, but it is within as great as yf they burned, wt moch heuynesse of the head, drynesse of þ mouth, & extreme thirste. Wherby many one are cōpelled for to slepe euen for very labour of the spirytes, and some other watche, and are so out of quyete that a man wolde thynke they were fallen in to a phrensye.

¶ The fourth signe is, yf great vapours
and

the pestilence.

and fumes aryse out of the body, when a man is in a bathe, and wolde fayne sweate, but he can not.

The fyfth sygne is yf the pacyent can not drawe hys breath;e easelye, for many one is so strayte wynded, that he can not speake, and when he breatheth it is with great labour and difficultie.

The syxt sygne is vehement payne of the heed, suche as is wont to be in a frenesye. But there be some for all that that in the begynnyng of the infection, fele nothing so great peyne as we haue spoken of in the heed. Notwythstandynge this is a general rule, ȝ the pestilence can not be in the body, withoute some payne, or heuynesse, in the heed.

The .vii. signe is great desyre to slepe, from the whyche many one can not abstayne hym selfe in anye wyse, nor can not be kept wakinge of them that are about hym.

The .viii. sygne is chaungynge of the syght, for somtymes there commeth to the pacientes eyes, as it were a yelowe colour,

A treatyse of

colour, somtymes all that he beholdeth he thynketh it to be grene.

The .ix. signe is peine of ẏ mouth, or an vnnatural tast, bytter, soure, or stiking

The tenth sygne is often vomytyng, bytter, and of dyuers colours.

The .xi. is heuynesse and dulnesse of al the hole body, and swownynge, and weakenesse of the lymmes. These be ẏ principal signes and tokens wherby ye may perceyue whē any man is infected.

Notwithstanding al these signes are not euer manifest, for somtymes it is sene, that one hath had the pestilence, & felt nothyng at all, yea and somtymes the vrine wyll be as fayre and as good to syght, as in a hole man, bycause the humours come not at the lyuer, and the feuer wylbe small or none, for that the venime is not in a hote humour, and so driueth out no heate, and yet the paciēt by and by dyeth.

Somtymes also he shall thynke hym self hole, bycause that nature in ẏ fyrst brunt draue the venyme from the hert,

and

the pestilence.

and yet anon after his lyfe passeth frō hym, for that nature was not strong ynough at the next assaute, eyther by reson it was vexed and weried in ye first, or els the venyme peraduenture multiplyed or chaunged in to more malignitie or nerer to the hert thā it was afore.

Euery one in the begynnynge seme lyghtly to be better for then the strēgth of nature is gathered all togyther to stande against his enemye, but it is not so in other euyll sycknesses. The paciēt also manye tymes thynketh hym selfe stronge ynoughe, bycause the venyme worketh not so cruellye vpon the other membres as it doth vpon the herte.

Wherfore in tyme of pestilence, when ye fele your selfe in any thyng diseased dryue not forth ye tyme in lokyng whē the signes aforesayd shuld appeare, nor stande not in crampnyng or doubtynge whether ye be isected or no, for ye may be sure, that so longe as thys dysease raygneth in the countrye where ye are, ye shall haue fewe sycknesses, but eyther

A treatyse of

ther is pestilence alreadye, or els wyll be within a whyle, and so gyue youre selfe to the cure of the Pestylence, for whyle the noughtye influence of that infection dureth, all superfluous humours maye lyghtly be enfected, and þ is the onelye cause, why in tyme of pestilence, there is so fewe of other infirmities.

For as soone as many sortes of other sykneſſes doo aryſe, the pestylence abateth and is gone.

And here is to be noted, that whatsoeuer chylde in the tyme of pestilence, be vexed with the wormes, ye may safelye affirme that he is infected, for it is a matter so disposed to the pestylence, euen as is brymstone, to be kyndled of the fyre. This haue manye phisitions not cōspired, and bicause of that, haue bene deceyued in theyr cure.   Here I haue declyned by occasion, but nowe to our intent.

When one or two, or more of these sygnes aforesayde are knowen to be in a
bodye

bodye, let hym not despyse them, nor put any foolysth trust in the strēgth of hys cōplexiō, as many one haue done, & by and by dyed, nor let no man trust ye colour of his vryne, or mouynge of the pulse: for sometymes the strength is so excessyue in the venyme, that a man is deed afore the naturall vertues are able for to succour hym, or to dryue awaye the venyme from the herte. And herein haue many wyse phisitions also ben deceyued, and haue euyll iudged of the pacientes pronostyke.

¶ Therfore by and by wythoute delaye, ye muste admynystre some good and holesome medycyne, as shalbe sayd hereafter, or elles the styled water that we spake of in the former Chapiter, or some other valyaunte medicine agaynst the pestylence, that it maye descende vnto the hert afore the venyme, haue the vpperhande of nature.

For yf it be ones settled at the hert, I affyrme playnely, there is no hope at al Yet there be some fooles, that tarye

A treatyse of

týl the twelueth houre, oz the foure and twentye after the infection, and they boost them selues that they wyll heale the pacient, but that is a manifeste and a shameful errour, for yf any by chaūce is so recouered, it commeth of God, & not of any medicyne, for where as one so escapeth, an hundred other peryshe.

Notwithstandynge yf the case so be that ye be not called, or can gette no remedye afore the sayde tyme, caste not your selfe into dispayre, or put not the paciēt in discomfort, take or gyue your medicine in the name of God, and yf ye can not brooke it, take as moche agayne & do so somany tymes tyll ye maye retayne it, then laye ye downe to sweate, and lyft vp your hert to God, callynge vpon him, without whome there is no helth, and by the grace of Iesu, ye nede not to be fearefull of deathe, for that þ is impossyble to man, is easye ynoughe with God, yea many times nature worketh it selfe, aboue all natural expectation. But I counsayl at the first begyn
nynge

the pestilence.

nynge to receyue the medicynes, when any of the forsayde sygnes appeareth, or when ye fele your selfe diseased, for the venyme perceth soner to the herte, of the cholerybe then either of the sanguyne or the melancholyke, althoughe the sanguynes are apter to infection, then the other are, chefelye yf the sycknesse be in somer.

They that are of melancholy be not lyghtly taken, but in case they be, then the cure is very daūgerouse and hard.

Therfore I saye take hede at the begynnyng as the prouerbe is.
Pūcipiis obsta, sero medicia paratur.
Cū mala per longas inualuere moras.

Take the medicine quyckly, and let thy selfe blood, and remembre God the phisicyon of thy soule, and wythoute doubt, thou shalt well ynough recouer.

Nowe we haue declared the sygnes by whych ye maye easely knowe when a persō is infected, and we sayd it was conuenient to take þ medicine as soone as any of thē appeareth, without any

P.ii. longer

A treatyse of

longer taryeng afore ẏ venyme cōmeth to the hert, here we wyl enfourme you, how ye shall perceyue whether the sayd venyme be settled in the hert or no.

☞Take a dramme of bolearmeny made in pouder accordyng to the doctrine of ẏ last chapter in ẏ fyrst parte, and yf ye can not get it, take some other excellent medicine agaynst the pestilence, namely one of the receptes that shall be sayde hereafter, and gyue it to the paciēt, but there can nothynge be better, then the foresayde pouder yf ye haue it at hand.

☞Take I say therof one dramme, and an ounce of whyte wyne and odoriferous, with two ounces of water of roses, myngle them, and gyue tyem to the pacient. The blacke recepte declared in the Chapiter of preseruatyues maye be well vsed in stede of the bole.

And yf he maye retayne the drynke within his stomacke, it is a good sygne that the venyme was not at the hert afore he toke the medicyne, and therfore he maye be let blood well ynough.

But

the pestilence

But yf the pacyent can not broke the said drynke, but cast it vp and vomyte, then ye may by sure, that the venymme hath ben at the hert afore the medicine

Therfore by and by wash his mouth with wine, or with water of scabiouse, of sorell, or of roses, and it ought to be very well mundifyed and clensed.

Then gyue hym an other dose of the sayd drynk, & heate a crust of bred, and holde it to his nose, that he may þ better kepe the forsayd pocion. And yf the second tyme he cast it vp agayne, and is not able to receyue it, wash his mouthe as is sayd before, and gyue it hym the thyrde tyme, wyth a lytle vynegre, þ it maye perce the better, and so vi. or. vii. tymes, yf he do not holde it, gyue it him agayne, and then whether he retayneth it, or reteyneth it not, by & by ye ought to let hym blood.

But in case the pacient were infected xxiiii. houres afore ye gyue the drynke, neuer let him blood, for that can nothig helpe hym, but rather make hym feble,

P.iii. but

A treatyse of

but admynystre a medicyne ordeyned for the pestylence, as is sayde afore, or such as shalbe spoken of hereafter, and that done prouoke hym to sweate.

Nowe to oure purpose as concernynge dyete.

❡ The seconde Chapter, of the cure of pestilence, by the way of diete.

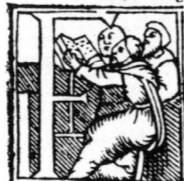

Fyrst as soone as euer the paciēt feleth hym self ifected, it is very good to auoide the corrupt ayer, by chaūgyng into some other place, or els yf he can not so, let him rectify the ayer of his owne house, or of his chambre, wyth water of roses & vyneger, or elles with fumigations as is spoken of before, accordynge to the qualitie of the tyme, and the complexiō of his owne bodye.

Moreouer it is good for him to shiften hys bedde out of one chambre into another,

the pestilence.

another, & from that to the fyrst agayne the next daye, euer rectifyng the ayer, of them both, as is afore sayd.

And as touchynge meate & drynke, he ought not to abstayne, nor yet to take any superfluities, for to eate good meates measurablye (though it be agaynste hys stomak) yet in this disease it shall do hym muche good: Lette him eate the broth of chyckyns, capons, or colepses of rabbetes, & suche lyke meates, with a lytle sorel sauce, or vinegre, and rosewater, or wyne of pomegranades, (yf they maye be gotten) or wyne of barberyes, and suche other.

If ye wyll haue other kynde of sauces, or a pouder to strowe vppon your meate, ye maye make it after thys sort.

Take graynes of paradyse, whyte dyptanye, of eche an ounce, fyne poudre of cynamome, and cloues, of eche halfe an ounce, make them all in poudre, and myngle it wyth suger. In thys disease ye maye eate no quesy meates, as eles, gese, duckes, & other suche as be euyll.

P.iiii.　　I call

A treatyse of

I call them euyll meates, whyche (accordyng vnto Galene De differentiis febrium) are eyther euyll of theyr owne nature, or els yf they be naturallye good, yet by reason of some putrefaction, are as muche or more vnholsome, as the other are, partlye so, bycause of longe kepynge vncleane and naughty dressinge, or when they be layed vp in a fylthy or stynking place, and partly by some yll infection, when they were alyue, for he that vseth such kynd of meates, is oftentymes accombred wyth manye naughtye syckenesses, as corrupte and pestilenciall feuers, scabbes, pustles, lepryes, and other euyl infirmities.

All fyshe in thys case are to be auoyded. Brothe or gruell, made wyth borage, buglosse, endyue, succorye, sorell, purcelane, and other lyke herbes, with a litle saffron, and cleane wheate flour, or ỹ cromes of bread in a broth of chyckyns, or wythout a broth, maye be wel admynistred,

Potched

the pestilence.

Potched egges also wyth sorel sauce and cinamome, vinegre and rosewater, are merueylous good in this case.

And yf the heate, be very vehement, as well after meate, as afore, he maye wel drynke a draught of sodden water with the iuyce of orenges, lymons, citrons, or of sowre apples, wel myngled togyther, to quenche the venymous fumes, that myght ryse vp to the brayne.

And yf the patient be yonge, & strong hauinge a good stomack, hole winded, hoote of complexion, and in tyme of heate, not subiecte to the colicke, nor to none hydropsie, nor apostemes in ye bowelles, he maye drinke a good draught or two of cleare and colde water comminge out of a rocke, or of a runninge water, or of a fayre sprynge. For when nothinge elles can mitigate the thirste, yet will cleare water by litle and litle, diminysh all the heate. But ye must beware ye take no great excesse.

A ptisane with suger of roses, is verye good to drynke betwene meales.

The

A treatyse of

The patient ought not for to sleape durynge the fyrst .xxiiii. houres, and in the tyme that he receyueth his medicines. Afterward he may slepe a little at ones, to comforte the weakenesse of the spyrytes, and he ought euery daye to go to syege ones.

And aboue all other thynges let him not dyspayre, but bidde hi be of good comforte, and doubt not of his health, so he take no thoughte, but as muche as is possible, make hym to reioyse, as well by communication as by musyke, and bryngynge in vnto hym good and holsome herbes, frutes, boughes, & other thinges of comfort, but yet notwithstādyng se that he remembrs God, and not forget his owne conscience, for in this sickenesse the worst is euer to be feared.

⁂ The thyrde chapter, of
the cure of pestilence
by the waye
of medi-
cine.

As

the pestilence.

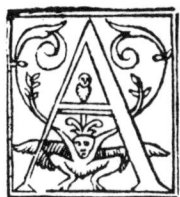

As soone as euer ye fele your selfe ifecte, take of the poudre of bole armoniake, in maner & fourme afore declared, or of ye blacke receyte the weyghte of halfe a crowne more or lesse accordyng to the vertue of the patient, myngled wyth the water of roses, and a lytle vynegre, as is sayde afore, and drynke it all at one draught.

And yf ye can not gette the forsayde pouder, or peraduéture ye wyll abhorre to take it, thē drink a litle potiō of ye receyte folowing, whyche is very excellēt.

⁋ A receyte agaynst the pestilence.

Take the rote of turmētile dryed in the shadowe, of saffron, and of mustard seede asmuch of one as of an other, make of them a poudre, and incorporate it wyth the thyrde parte of mithridatum, or of fyne triacle, wyth a lytle stronge vinegger,

A treatise of

ger, in maner of an opiate, kepe in an earthen vessell close, & in tyme of nede, vse it. The weight of it at ones is from halfe a dramme vpwarde.

Thys receyte woorketh more vpon the venime then it doth vpon the feuer. And euery daye folowyng it is good to take a litle sirupe of limons, wyth water of sorel, or of matfelon, or of our ladye thystell.

And he that hathe none of the sayde sirupes, let hym vse the waters of the same herbes, or the good water that I haue described in the Chapter of medicynes preseruatyues.

Auicenne sayth that who soeuer tasketh an onyon and drynketh it in mylke fasting in a morning he shal be safe that day from al infections of the pestilence Therfore some are wont to rost two or thre onyons, & to eate them wyth vinegre and browne breade nexte their hart afore they enter into any suspecte ayer. And haue founde health in their so doinge,

Johānes

the pestilence.

Ohánes Manardus, a man of hye knowledge in the art of medicine, and of greate auctoritye amonges al learned men, describeth in hys booke of Epistles, a very good receyte aswel preseruatyue as curatiue deuised by hym selfe for lacke of good triacle, and is of marueylous operation, as wel in this disease, as in healing all maner venymous woundes, both of adders, snakes, and other kinde of serpentes. The receyte of thys noble medicine is this.

¶ Mainardus medicine for
the pestilence.

Ake the dryed bloode of a drake, and of a ducke, of a gose, and of a kyd, rue, fenel seede, the seede of cumyne, dylle, and of wylde nepes, or gardē nepes, or rapes, of euerye one thre drāmes, of the roote of gētiane, trifoyle, squinantum, franken sence, roses dryed, of eche. iiii. drammes Whyte peper and longe, coste, valerian
any se

A treatyse of

anyse, cynamome, of eche two drammes myrrhe, narde, of eche vi. drames, bensiamin, assarum, gumme armoniake, of eche thre drammes, aloes, agaryke, of eche two drammes, carpobalsami, xx. graynes, preos, saffron, reubarbe, and reupontyke, gynger, mastyke, of eche one dramme, sticados, fyue drammes.

Make a fyne pouder of these, and with foure tymes as moch of claryfyed honye, myngle all togyther, and kepe it in a syluer vessel or a glasse stopped, for it is an hye treasure, in such a case. The dose of it is two drammes in wyne or water of sorell.

¶ Here foloweth an electuarye of a wonderful vertue in the tyme of pestilence.

This electuarye is of so greate vertue, in that they do receyue it, ones in xviii. houres, that they maye be sure from all euyll infections of corrupte ayres, and contagyous all the daye after.

But in them that are enfecte alreadye

the pestilence.

dye, and are taken wyth the pestilence, yf they drynke of it but one sponefull, as shall be sayde hereafter, (specyally after lettynge bloode yf it be conuenient to the patient) and laye hym downe and sweate vppon the same, yf the venyme hathe not vtterlye ouercome the harte, he shall vndoubtedlye recouer. It hath bene latelye proued, that after drynkynge of the same medicine whan the patiēt made his water in an vrinal the glasse hath broste in pieces, by reason of the venyme that it purged out.

¶ Thys is the makyng of the sayde electuarye.

Take cynamome electe one ounce, terra sigillata. vi. drāmes, fyne myrrhe thre drāmes, vnicornes horne. i. drāme the seede and rynde of citron, rootes of diptany, burnet, turmentylle, zedoarie, redde corall, ana, drammes ii. yelowe saunders. iiii. scruples, red saunders, ii. scruples, whyte ben and redde, floures of marygoldes, ana, one dramme, yuerye raced, scabiouse, beroniel tunies, seede

A treatyse of

seede of basile, ye bone of a stagges hart saffron. ana. ii. scrupules, make a fyne poudre, and adde vnto it of bole armoniake preparate. ii. ounces, white suger iii. pounde, and with a syrupe of accositate citri, make a goodlye electuarye, and kepe it in a glasse.

If the pestilence commeth wt greate excesse of heate, drinke it vpon rosewater, and vynegre, but yf ye fele it colde, take it in a draught of wyne, and couer ye, wyth clothes, so that ye may sweate as longe as is possible, for wythoute doute, it is a presente remedie as I my selfe haue oftentymes proued.

⁋ An other deuyne medecyne, in a lyquyde fourme.

The rewe, woormewood & bawme ye herbe, of eche a lyke portion, of celidonye, bothe herbe & rote, as moche as al ye other, so yt ye haue of them foure, a good bigge hadeful, wasshe ye rote of celidonye

the pestilence.

lidonye, very clene and purely, in wine or in fayre clere water, than put them all into a newe pot of earth nelod with in, and poure vppon the herbes, halfe a pounde of the moste strongest vynegre, ye can gette, couer them iuste, and lute the mouth of the potte, wyth luto sapiencie, whiche is made of wheate floure and the whyte of an egge, that no breth maye issue, and seethe it .viii. or .ix. houres, wyth a softe fyer, than let it coole be lyttle and lytle, and after strayne the herbe, and set the lycoure in the sonne to rectifye.

¶ Whan person is infected with the pestilence, Fyrste as I sayde afore, let hym bleede in a due vayne, than gyue hym a sponefull of this lycoure, wyth as moche as a nutte of tryacle, yf so be ye haue any, luke warme, by and by let a cruste of bread all hote, be dypped in vynegre, and holden to hys mouth, that he may the better brooke the medicine.

And yf he chaunce to vomyte, incontynent wasshe hys mouth wyth wyne,

A treatyse of

and cause hym to receyue agayne an other sponeful, & so yf nede be. v. oz. vi. tymes, tyl ye se that he reteyne it, whyche is a verye good sygne, yf he so do.

After this set hym in a warme bed couered, that he maye sweate out the resydue of the venyme, and by the grace of God, he shall escape the daunger. Thys is a medieyne of infinite vertue. But if the payent haue a great heate gyue hym no tryacle, oz elles verye litle,

⁋ The .iiii. chapter of the cure of pestilence, by lettynge of blood, ventoses, and purgations.

Although phlebotomye oz lettyng of blood, be one of the chyefe thinges that are requyred to the cure of the pestylence, yet foz lacke of vnderstandynge & lettynge blood, otherwyse than behoueth, manye one is cast awaye, and therefoze euerye good barbour

the pestylence.

bour ought for to take heed, ꝑ he hurte not them, whyche come vnto hym for helpe, (for that were a greatte shame) whyche he shall neuer do, yf he ponder wel ꝑ thynges, ꝑ shal be sayd hereafter.

¶ Thys is a general rule.

An ꝑ tyme of pestilēce whan a bodye is infect ye may not haue respect eyther to the sygne, ꝑ day or ꝑ houre, but whether ꝑ mone be there, or nto, or what aspectes so euer be in the planettes lette hym blede forth with in the name of God.

Younge men and sanguine, and they that haue aboundaunce of flesshe, and of blood mingled wyth other humors, ought to blede somewhat more in quā titye, but alwayes kepe a moderation, that ye take not oute to great a quanti tye at ones.

It is better to let hym blood twyse leuynge the wonde of the fyrst stroke open, and anoynt it wyth a lytle ople, and after foure or fyue hou:res, let hym

D.ii. blede

A treatyse of

blede in the same wounde agayne, but wythout strykyng yf it be possyble.

But allwayes gyue an eye, to the strengthe of the paciente, that it be not enfebled, and agayne beware that ye haue taken awaye the rankest, and the strongest venyme, wherin yf ye be dout full, take the counsayle of some good expert phisition.

Also ye muste note, that ye maye not let bloode, to any chyldren wythin the age of. xiiii. yere, nor to olde men about fyftye yere olde, nor to women greatte wyth chylde specially nere vnto theyre tyme, nor when theyre due purgations is vpon them, nor to them þ are newely brought to bed, or wtin a weke. or. if. after she is puryfied, generallye to none whych is weake & feble in hys bodye.

Ye shall also note, that there are some olde menne of better strength and complexion, than manye yonge are of, and agayne dyuers younge chyldren of ten or twelue yeres olde, are of hygher co-tage, and of as good strength, as theye
that

that are manye yeres elder. In such cases, a lytle euentation of the enfected bloode, maye be the sauynge of theyre lyues, so that all thynges be done with good discretion.

It is wysdome also to let the blood lyenge vppon theyr backes whome ye thynke woulde faynte in standynge or in syttynge.

And yf the case do requyre the lettynge of blood, and the pacient be not able to beare it for any of the causes afore rehersed, it is good to applye ventoses, in maner and fourme as I shall declare hereafter.

And here we shulde saye somwhat of the great errour that many do commyt in takynge one veyne for an other, for by suche errours is the venym drawen manye tymes vnto the herte, and so procureth deathe vnto the pacient.

Wherefore that ye maye not be disceyued, euer in the pestilence lette hym bloode on that syde that the sore is on, and not on the contrarye syde, in anye wyse,

A treatyse of

wyse, for that shulde drawe the venim ouerthwarte the membres spirytuall, and so destroye the man.

But or euer ye lette hym blood, it is good to gyue some good, and holsome medicine agaynste the venyme, such as is declared in the chapters herebefore.

If the botche appere vnderneth the eares, let him blood in the hed veyne of the same arme, or els in the braunche of the same venyme, whyche is vpon the hande, betwene the myddle fynger and the nexte that is adioynyng.

If it appeare vnder the throte, take the same veyne, & wythin a whyle after, it is good to open the .ii. veynes vnderneth the tongue.

If the sore be sette wythin the arme holes, take the veyne called mediana, whyche is betwene the soresayd heade veyne, and the veyne commynge from the lyuer.

If the sore be sette wythin the flankes, than he muste open the veyne called saphena, whyche is about the ancle

of

the pestilence.

of the fote, on the inner syde, and yf ye can not fynde it there, take the branch of it, that is betwene the great too, and the nexte vnto hym, but the lettynge of bloode in that veyne is forbydden vnto women when they be in health.

And yf there apere. ii. botches, one on euery syde, Manardus gyueth councell to take the ryght syde and not the lyft.

And in case ther doth appere no signe of botche or swellyng, than he biddeth you to open bothe the veines saphenas on the ryght syde and the lefte.

Notwythstadynge Marsilius Ficinus is of a cōtrarie opinion & sayeth that it is beste when there doth no sore appere, to take the cōmon veyne one of the ryght arme.

I thynke herein manardus councell rather to be folowed.

But yf ye se y botche standyng out warde more towarde the bounche, than ye muste open the veyne called sciatica, whyche is aboute the ancle of the fote on the outsyde. The whyche opnynge

D. iiii. of the

of the veynes muste be done as sone as is possyble, alwaye presupposed, that he hath receyued one or other medicine agaynste the venym, and that he sleape not in any wise, as is afore mentioned.

And to them that can not lawfullye be letten blood, ye muste in all haste applye many ventoses, with scarification or wythout scarifienge, as it seameth beste to your discretion, so ye take a reasonable order thus, If the sore be vnder the eares, or about the throte, lette youre ventoses be applyed behynde vpon the necke.

If þ botche appeare vnder þ armes set your ventoses behynd vpon þ shulders

If the sore be in the flanke, or thyes, lette youre ventoses be sette vppon the buttockes.

And yf the patiente be replete wyth humours and stronge, hauyng no flure nor other impedimente, & ye thynke he nedeth to be purged, ye maye gyue hym in þ mornyng .i. ounce of cassia, or of mãna, w a litle dyaprunis laxatyue, more or lesse,

the pestilence.

or lesse, according to the pacients necessity tempered wt water of scabiouse, sorell, or endiue, euer taking hede, that he do receyue some medicyne agaynst þ venym during al the tyme of hys discase.

¶ The fyfthe Chapiter of applycation of outewarde medicines.

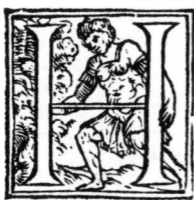

Ere is to be noted that no maner playster repercussiue, maye be set vppon any botch of pestilence. But assoone as is possyble, after lettyng blood, it is good to take an onion, and to make an hole in þ middest of it, then fyll it full of good tryacle, after that stoppe it, and set it on the harthe to roste, as it were an apple. And when it is roste so longe tylle it be tendre, let it cole a lytle: and set it hote vpon the botche, and when it hath ben there by the space of two houres, take
there

A treatyse of

it of, and laye an other on.

Or take, a cocke and pull the fethers of, aboute hys foundament, & put a little salt in it, and set his foundament vppon the sayde botche, kepyng hym on a good whyle, stopppng many tymes hys byll, that his breth may be reteyned, & let hym blowe agayne. And yf the cocke die, it shalbe good to take another yong cocke, and sp'ytte it quycke asounder, & lay it on ye botche, but ye must cōmaūde them that take them of, to cast them in ye fyre, & not to take the sauour whē it is remoued: for that is very daūgerous

Some there be that laye aboute the sore, water leches called bloodsuckers, and it is very good, so they be well prepared, and clensed, from corruption.

Other apply ventoses wyth scarificatiō, but they ought fyrst to be applied wythouten anye scarifyng, so they shal the better drawe the venyme out.

Other lay therto a playster made of galbanū, diaquilō, & armoniake, incorporate togyther, & some other lay on it
a plaister

the pestilence.

a plaister made of figges soure leuen, & reisins without kernels, brayed & icorporate all togyther in oyle of camomylle. There be also that set vpon þ botche an herbe called crowefoote, whiche is very hoote, and maketh a blyster on the skynne, and that same they breake, and kepe the place open many dayes after. And in that case, yf the botche be in the very arme holes: it is beste to set þ sayd herbe a lofte vpon the arme.

And some other breake the forsayd botche wyth a strong ruptory, hauyng part of maturatiō, as for exāple thus.

Take sowre leuen, foure ounces, mustarde, rue, scabiouse, wormewood, of euery one an handefull, whyte lylly rotes, the thyrde parte of all, greene coppotose two drammes, cantharides in numbre. x. galbani one ounce, olde nuttes, and somwhat fusty, or els newe yf ye can not get thē, in numbre. iiii. oyle of whyte lilies, as moch as shal suffyce, seeth all the herbes and rootes in oyle, accordynge to arte, wyth a double vessel,

A treatise of

el that is to saye: the oyle beyng in one panne maye sethe onely by the boylyng of ẏ water in an other greatte panne, and make a playster wyth the respdue of the stuffe in a good fourme. It hath a great vertue to breake a pestilēce sore wythoute moch payne, and afore ye lay it on, wasſh the sore wyth a sponge dip ped in the straynynge of the foresayde herbes and rotes.

Other take oyle olyue and seth it with oken asſhes, addynge vnto it a lytle of blacke sope, and quicke lyme, and make a playster of the same, it is not to be v- sed, but in strong complexions.

And al ẏ forsayd wayes are to be com- mended. But after one hath vsed thē a whyle, & seeth they begynne to come to maturation, let him take ẏ counsell of a lerned surgeon, or any other of good experience, and to set maturatyue em- playsters, vnctions, and bathes, accor- dynge as beeſmeth, peryng the apo- steme in the softeste place, afterwarde procede wyth mundification and incar

nation

nation, euen as in other kyndes of appostemes, wherein I humblye desyre them to haue some pytye of the poore, that be diseased, & not to fauoure them that haue ynough, but rather take somoch of the rych þ they may the better haue wherwyth to helpe the nedye.

And for bycause the sycke may haue some cōfort, if in case they shulde be destitute of surgeons, I wyl(besydes the said medicines which they may cōfidētlye vse,)describe some maturatiue emplayster that are expert and proued in this cure of pestilēce.

⁋ A playster to rype a botche cōmynge of the pestilence.

Take mallowes, & the rotes of holyhocke, & onions, asmuch as shall suffice, waste them & seeth them in water, and afterwarde bray them i a morter with poudre of lineseed, & of fenugreke, & a good quantitie of swines grese fresh, laying on the playster euery day ones.

⁋ An other for the same

Take

A treatyse of

The white diptany an ounce and an halfe, the rote of walwort an ounce, the rootes of cresses halfe an ounce, whyte onyons .ii. onces, seeth the rotes in water, and rost the onion vpon the coles, then stampe them al togyther, addynge of oyle of camomill .iii. ounces, rosyn one ounce, nettle seede syre drãmes, waxe, asmuch as shal suffice, and make a goodlye playster or an oyntinēt at your pleasure, for it ripeth the sayde botche in a shorte space & consumeth the venyme, and is good aswell for yonge men as for olde.

And afore that it be thorough rype, cause it to be perced as it is sayd afore. And yf after the sayde percing there be greate payne, take the yolke of an egge well beaten, and a lytle oyle of roses, & annoynte a tent therin, and put into y sore, for to cease the payne. Afterwarde mundifye the place wyth a salue made of yolkes of egges, fyne barly floure, & a lytle hony of roses. Laste of al, for the perfecte incarnation, take the iuyce of
daysies,

the pestilence.

dayses, and wyth a lytle waxe make a softe oyntment, & vse it, or ye maye laye therto anye other salue incarnatyue, as ye are wont to do in other clene sores.

Prouyded alway that it is better in this case, to breake the sore betymes than to tarye for the ryppyng long, least perchaunce the venym beyng included, gather strength by the putrefaction, & so returne agayne vnto the harte, therfore open it, afore it come to ryppynge, & after procede with your maturatyues, and other holsome playsters.

Thus moche haue I spoke of surgerye, in the exterior cure of one that hath the botche, so farre as god hath giuen me vnderstandynge to perceyue, accordyng to the mindes of suche famouse clerkes, as haue moste effectually wrytten on the same. Nowe wyll I declare a lytle of the exterior cure of hym that hath no botche at all, and yet is sore infected with the pestilence. For the noble handy woorke of surgery, is conueniēt to them bothe, as

wytnesseth

A treatyse of
wytnesseth Marsilius Ficinus, in his booke of pestilence in the .xi. Chapiter. And the fourme of it is thys.

After that the pacient hath receyued some good & holsome medicyne against the pestilence, and swette (or after lettynge blood, yf the case do so requyre) by and by ye must apply your labour to take awaye the residue of the venyme, that remaineth i the body. And to that intent ye oughte to make a ruptorie of sowre leuen & cantharides, or other aboue rehersed, & set it on the muscule, of the ryght arme, vnder the cubyte, on the parte, where as the pulse lyeth, but not vppon the pulse it selfe, and so procure a blystre, whiche ye shall immediatly cut of, & kepe the sore runnyng many dayes after, the longer the better for the pacient.

An other issue ye maye make in the same maner, vpon his right legge, four fingers aboue his heele toward the insteppe, and kepe it open lykewyse, tyl a moneth or two after he be recouered.

℃ The

the pestilence

⁋ The .vi. Chapiter, of the cure of
carbuncles and anthrax.

COncernynge the curation both of a carbuncle & the pestilence sore called anthrax, ye maye do euerye thynge accordynge as we spake afore in the general cure of the pestilence, both as touching diete, medicynes agaynste the venyme, cordialles, laxatyues, blood lettynges, and ventoses, ye shall heale them as ye heale the botche, in al thynges.

But as touchynge lettynge bloode, when ye se a carbuncle or an anthrax by hym selfe wythout aposteme of the emunctoryes, be it vpon the necke, or vppon the throte, or the face, or the heade, ye must let him blood in the head veyne

If it be vpon the shoulders, brestes, or arme or other place aboue the naupl, take the veyne called mediana.

And yf it be beneth the sayde places, downe vnto the knees, take the veyne sephena, but yf it be on the outsyde of the thygh, take the veyne sciatica, euer

R.i.   vpon

A treatyse of

vpon the syde that the sore is on,(as is sayde afore)consyderyng the complexion, the strength, the age, and the qualitie of the blood, euen as it is said in the chapter of the botche, and lykewise applye the ventoses vppon them that can not beare flebothompe.

Whyche thynges presupposed it is good to set vpon the carbūcle, whether it be with botche or without botch, the yolke of an egge, incorporate wyth as much sa't as ye can tēper with it, renuyng it euery houre duryng a hole daye.

Or els apply the said leches or blood suckers rounde aboute the sore, & after they haue sucked out $ bloode, set theron a cocke as is said of the botch, or els a doue al hote splytte in the myddle.

And he that can not gette the leches, yet let hym not fayle to apply the resydue of the sayde medicynes, euerye one after other as afore is sayd.

Or a hote lofe commynge out of the ouen, or take a sower pomgranade, and cut and seeth it in vinegre, or scabious
brused

of the veynes.

brused betwene two stones, or ye rote of dayses, or good sowre dough, incorporate wyth salte and a lytle oyle olyue, al these medicines are good to kyll the carbuncle.

The preciouse stone called a saphyre hath also great vertue against venyme and specially agaynst a carbuncle, if ye towche it wt the stone, & drawe it rounde aboute ye sore by ye space of an houre.

But what soeuer medicine ye set vnto a carbuncle, ye must laye a defensiue about the sore, whyche is made as here after foloweth.

¶ A good defensyue.

Take sanguis draconis, & bole armeny, of eche a like much, make them in pouder & incorporate them wt ople of roses, & a lytle vynegre, & laye it in a clothe all about the sore, wout touchig any part of it, & renewe it when it is hard & dry.

But yf the person be of good abilitie & the carbuncle very fearce & burnyng, can not be quenched wyth the meanes aforesayde, than ye muste procede with
R.ii.   an

A treatise of

an actuall oꝛ potentiall cauterie, and to remoue the escare, lay on capons grece oꝛ a lytle butter, oꝛ els a playster made of mallowe leaues, holihockes, violettes, lyly rotes sodden in bꝛoth of netes fete oꝛ other flesshe, and afterward stāped, streyned, & vpon the fyer myngled with pouder of lyneseede, barly floure beane floure, fresshe butter, and swines grece, addyng in the ende whan ye take it of, two yolkes of egges and a lytle saffron, and styꝛre it well aboute.

This is good also to rype the foꝛsaid soꝛe, afterwarde mundifye & heale as is sayde in the other chappter.

I coulde declare many other remedies but I set them ꝑ haue be often pꝛoued, and ꝑ be moste easye foꝛ to get at nede, desyꝛynge all them that shall vse these my simple labours, to accepte my good wyl vnto the best, and to pꝛaye to God almyghtye foꝛ hys grece, vnto whome onlye be al laude, gloꝛye and honoure, woꝛlde wythoute ende. Amen.

¶A declaration of the

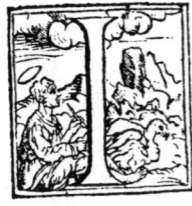

veynes in mannes bodye,
and to what dyseases,
and infyrmytyes
the o=
penynge of euerye one
of them do
serue.

¶Tis not vnkno=
wen to any whi=
che haue sene A=
nathomyes, how
there be in a man
nes body. ii. kyn=
des of veynes ge=
nerall and speci=
all.

¶Generalle or commune veynes are. iii. whyche appere in the myddeste of e=
uery mannes arme on the inner syde, & of them the highest is called of learned mē cephalica, or the head veyne and the loweste of all thre, is called commonly

A.iii. basi=

¶ declaracion

basilica oʒ regia, in the ryght arme by an other name epatica, oʒ the veyne of the lyuer, but in the lyft arme, it is called pulmatica, the veyne of the longes.

¶ The .iii. cōmon veyne, lyeth betwene the other .ii. in the myddes, and is named coʒdiaca, oʒ the veyne of the herte.

¶ The fyʒst that we dyd speke of, that is to saye cephalica, is a veyne most apt to be letten bloode, in all the hyer partes of mannes bodye, and is opened for the head ache, and the eyes.

¶ Thys veyne yf by chaunce ye touche it, and yf it blede not at the fyrst stroke ye may be bolde to stryke it ones agayn for there is no ieoperdye of cuttynge of anye muscle. And yf ye can not fynde it oute, take hys braunche that is aboute the thombes ende.

¶ The veyne epatica, emptyeth from the myddle partes of all the body, and it is euer opened agaynst dyseases of þ stomacke and the splene, but ye oughte therin to be verye dylygente, that there be no muscule perced.

If ye

of the veynes.

If ye can not spye it in the arme, seke the braunche of it betwene the lytle finger and the fourth.

The cordiaca veyne draweth blood as well from byneth, as from aboue for it is cōpouned of cephalica and epatica.

If any feleth a weaknes at his hart he oughte to take good hede that he be not opened in the veyne cordiaca, but if necessitie be of bledyng, lette him blede in the cephalica or els mediana. So lykewise of the other two. The cordiaca, is good to cure the passions of al the hole bodye, whan they do procede of heate, specially of the harte and of the longes.

But in the pereynge of it, ye must exceedyngly beware, for vnder it is a certayn muscule, which if it be very depely cutte, the pacient is in ieopardye of hys lyfe.

Whan ye entend to let a person blood in anye veyne, ye muste bathe the arme wherin ye perce, in good hote water, & drawe ȳ hole abrode, ȳ the grosse blood

R.iiii.   maye

of veynes.

may the more easely passe. And here is to be noted, that in all sikneſſes and tymes (except only infection of the peſtylence) ye muſte take the ſame veyne of the .iii. that doth appere fuller and bygger thā þ other are, for by that ye may perceyue that the membres whyche belong vnto it, are full of ſuperfluyties of to hote blood, and this ſhalbe ſufficient of the forſayde veynes generall, nowe we wil reherce þ veynes ſpecial.

⁋ The veyne ī the hygher part of the forehead, is good to be opened in al diſeaſes of the head, and of the brayne, ſpeciallye yf they be of longe continuance, and it cureth the newe begonne lepry.

⁋ The .ii. veynes that are behynde the eares, are opened to preſerue the memory, mundifie the face, and to take away reumes and diſtillations from þ heade and are good generallye in all dyſeaſes of the mouthe, and of the gummes

⁋ The .ii. veynes of the temples of the head, are good to voide humours from the eyes, and they ſerue alſo for all diſeaſes of vaynes.

eases of the eares.

The .ii. veynes in the corners of the eyes are opened in the cure of webbes, spottes, cloudes, mistes, perles, rednes comes, & other infirmities and weaknesse of the syght.

The .ii. veynes in the holowenes of the eares, serue to heale the shakyng of the head, swymmynge of the eyes, dosynes, soundyng of the eares, newe deafnesse, and vncleannes of the mouthe.

The veyne in the toppe of the nose, is good agaynste apostemes of the heade, reumes, and fluxes of the eyes, it pourgeth the brayne, and comforteth the memorye.

This veyne muste be soughte verye wysleye, for it lyeth depe, therfore he y̅ wyll be sure of it, shall fynde it euen in the verye myddes betwene the two sides of the nose ende.

The two veynes within the nosthrilles, are opened against the heuynesse of the head.

The veyne of the lyppes, is good to take

A declaration

take in all diseases of the mouth.

¶ The .ii. veynes within the mouth, are opened in diseases of the heed, toth ach payne of the iawes, mouth and throte, and agaynst freeles of the face.

¶ The foure veynes in the palate of the mouth, are good to be opened in toth ache, reumes and catarres of the heed.

¶ The two veynes in the hyndre parte of the heed, are good agaynste the phrenesye, swymmynge, astonyinge, and all other paynes of the heed.

¶ The .ii. veynes vnderneth the tõg are opened against þ flures of the heed, palsyes, quyncies, scrophules, apoplexia, cough, paynes of the mouth, teeth, and gummes agaynst impedimentes of the speche, and generally in all diseases of the breast, hert, longes and arteries.

¶ The veyne that is betwene the chyn, and the nether lippe, is good to open in curyng of a stynkyng breath.

¶ The veyne that lyeth ryght vnderneth the chynne, is good agaist þ same
disease,

disease, and also in diseases of the heed & of the brest, polipus in the nose, paynes of ye chekes, stinking of ye nosethrilles, scrophules & spottes about the face

❡ The two veynes of the necke (one afore, an other behynde) are excedynge good agaynste the pleuresye, newe lepzye, shakyng of the membres, humoures, and distillations of the heed, and to moche styfnes of lymmes.

❡ The two veynes vnder the arme holes, serue agaynst the straytnesse of the brest, payne of the mydryfe, and the lōges, and agaīst difficultie of breathing called asthma.

❡ The two veynes about the elbowes are taken in all dyseases of the breast, swymmyng of the heed, spasme, and epilepsia, cōmō'y called the fallyng eupl.

❡ Vena purpurea or the purple veyne, lyinge in the ryght arme nexte epatica, towarde the hande, is opened agaynste diseases of spirituall membres, and of the bowels.

❡ The veyne iliaca nexte vnto the purpyle

of vaynes.

ple veyne, yf it be well taken, is good to heale the paynes of all the inwarde membres.

¶ Vena pulsatilis, or the beatyng veine is good agaynste the tremblynge of the hert, swowpyng, and cardiaca passio.

¶ The .ii. veynes of the thumbes, are opened in diseases of the heed, bleared eyes, and agaynst the moost parte of al feuers.

¶ The veyne betwene the forefynger and the thombe, is good for stoppynge of the heed, and to purge the superfluitye of cholere, is good in agues, and in all diseases of the eyes.

¶ The veyne that is betwene the ryngfynger, and the lytle (yf it be opened) taketh awaye diseases of the heed, the longes, of the splene.

¶ The veine called saluatella in ye right hande, betwene the litle fynger and the next adioynynge, is opened in oppilations of the brest, against ye gumy matter of the eyes, perbrakynge, yelowe iaundys, paynes & colykes in the right syde

of

of the belly. And in the lefte hande it is opened against al diseases of the splene comyng of repletiō and oppilatiō, and is good to heale the hemoroides, phrenesye, colickes in the left syde, diseases of the veynes, and to moche aboūdaūce of the floures.

¶The veyne of the ryght syde, yf it be opened, is good in lienteria, dissuria, dropsyes and other infirmities caused of colde matter.

¶The veyne of the lefte syde is good agaynst apostemes and excoriations of the bladder, paynes of the loynes, swellyng and stoppyng of the splene.

¶The veyne of the bellye, is good agaynst diseases of the reynes, and purgeth out the melancholye blood.

¶The foure veynes about the place called pecten, on eyther syde the priuie mēbres, ar good agaist superfluous issues of the hemoroides, and to swage payne in all diseases of ẏ bladder, & the secret places, they stoppe the bledynge of the nose, & of other mēbres, and are good
to

A treatyse

to heale the lienterie and strangurye.

The veyne ouer the foreskynne of the yarde is opened agaynst the dropsy and all diseases of the same membre.

The veyne vnderneth the sayde skin is holsome to be taken for the crampe, or spasme, colyke, swellynge of the coddes, strangurye, dissurie, and dyseases of the stone, bothe in the reynes and in the bladder.

The two veines of the thyghes haue a singuler vertue in the curinge of dyseases in the bladder, and the reynes.

The two veynes in the legges, doo serue againste the dropsye, payne and a postemations of the bladder, and ye reynes, and the priuie membres, and against goute and swellyng of the knees.

The veyne saphena on the inner side of the legge, is opened agaynst retentiō of the flowres, and in all diseases of of the matrice, reynes, hyppes, pryuye places of men and wemen.

The outwarde saphena, otherwyse called sciatica, descending from the legges

A declaration

ges on the outſyde, is creeding good in curyng the payne of the huckle boone, whereof it hath the name ſciatica, and ouer that it healeth all diſeaſes of the bladder, and the bowels, goute of the handes and of the feete, wyth other payne of the ioyntes, and the palſye.

The two outwarde veynes vpon the ancles, are good to be opened for retention of the floures, they take awaye the ſwkneſſe of ÿ ſplene, and eaſe the payne of the backe, ſtranguric, and ſtone.

The two veynes vnder the lytle too, are good to purge the ſuperfluitye of the matryce, and to hele ſcrophules of the face and the legges.

The two veynes adioynynge to the lytle too, cure the apoplexie, yelowe cholere, palſye, and all diſeaſes of the reynes.

The .ii. veynes in the leſſer ioynt of the lytle too, are opened in curing of an olde cough, puſtles, and ophthalmia in the eyes,

The

A declaracion

The two veynes in the myddle too are good agaynste the scrophules, and diseases of the face, spottes, rednesse, and pymples, watryng of the eyes, cākers and knobbes, and agaynst the stoppyng of the floures.

The veyne on the left ioynte in the great too, is good agaynst ophthalmia of the eyes, spottes of the face and the legges, ytche, and ulcers of euyll complexion, and purgeth superfluities of the matrice.

Thus moche I haue declared of the vtilitie of veynes.

❡FINIS.

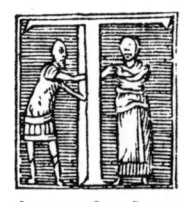

The boke of chyldren.

To begyn a treatyse of the cure of chyldren, it shulde seme expedyent, that we shuld declare somewhat of the pryncyples as of the generacion, the beinge in the wombe, the tyme of procedynge, the maner of the byrth, the byndyng of the naupll, settynge of the membres, lauatoryes, vnctions, swathinges, & entreatementes, with the circumstaunces of these and many other, which if I shuld reherce in particles, it wolde requyre both a longer tyme, and encrease into a greater volume. But forasmoch, as the moost of these thynges are verye trye & manifest: some pertayning onely to þ office of a mydwyfe, other for the reue-

The boke

tence of the matter not mete to be disclosed to euery vyle person: I entende in this boke to let them all passe, and to treate onely of the thynges necessarye, as to remoue the sycknesses, wherwith the tender babes are oftentymes afflycted, and desolate of remedye for so moche as manye do suppose that there is no cure to be ministred vnto them, by reasō of theyr weakenesse. And by that vayne opinion, yea rather by a foolyshe feare, they forsake manye that myght be well recouered, as it shall appeare by the grace of God hereafter, in thys lytle treatyse, when we come to declaration of the medicynes. In the meane season for confinitye of the matter, I entend to wryte somwhat of ye nource and of the mylke, wyth the qualities & complexions of ye same, for in that cōsysteth the chefe poynt and summe, not onelye of the mayntenaunce of healthe, but also of the fourmyn or infectyng eyther of the wytte, or maners, as the Poet Uergill when he wolde descrybe

an

an vncurteys, churlysh, and a rude con=
dichioned tyraunt, dydde attrybute the
faute vnto the gyuer of the mylke, as
in sayinge thus.

Nec tibi diua parens, generis nec Dar=
danus author.

Perfide, sed duris genuit te cautibus
horrens. Caucasus, hircaneq̄ admorūt
vbera tigres

For that deuyne Poet being through=
ly expert in the priuities of nature, vn=
derstode ryght well how great an alte=
ration euerye thynge taketh of the hu=
moure, by the whych it hathe his aly=
mēt & nourysyng in the youth: which
thyng also was conspyred and alleged
of manye wyse Philosophers: Plato,
Theophrastus, Xenophon, Aristotle, &
Plinie, who dydde all ascrybe vnto the
nourcement, as moche effect or more, as
to the generacyon.

And Phauorinus the Philosopher (as
wryteth Aulus gelius) affirmeth that if
lambes be nouryshed wyth the milke of
goates, they shall haue course wolle, lyke

lyke the heare of gootes, and of kyddes in lyke maner sucke vpon shepe, ẏ heare of them shalbe softe lyke wolle. Wherby it doth appeare, that the mylke and nouryshyng hath a maruevlous effecte in chaungyng the complexion, as we se lykewyse in herbes and in plantes, for let the seede or rympes by neuer so good and pure, yet yf they be put into an vnkynde earth, or watred with a noughty and vnholsome humour, eyther they come not vp at all, or els they wyll degenerate and turne out of theyr kynde, so that scarse it may appeare frō whēce they haue ben takē: accordig to ẏ verse.

Pomacg degenerant, succos oblita priores.

Wherfore as it is agreing to nature, so is it also necessary and comly for the owne mother to nource the owne child Whyche yf it maye be done, it shall be moost cōmendable and holsome, yf not ye must be well aduised in takyng of a nource, not of yll cōplexion & of worse maners: but suche as shall be sobre, honest

of chyldren.

nest and chaste, well fourmed, amyable and chearefull, so that she maye accustome the infant vnto myrthe, no dronkarde, vycyous nor sluttysh, for suche corrupteth the nature of the chylde.

But an honest woman (suche as had a man chylde last afore, is best) not within two monethes after her delyueraūce, nor approchynge nere vnto her tyme agayne. These thynges ought to be consydred of euery wyse person, that wyll set theyr chyldren out to nource.

Moreouer, it is good to loke vpon the mylke, & to se whether it be thycke and grosse, or to moche thynne and watrye, blackysshe or blewe, or enclynyng to rednesse or yelowe, for all suche are vnnaturall and euyll. Lykewyse when ye taste it in youre mouthe, yf it be eyther bytter, salte, or soure, ye may well perceyue it is vnholsome

That mylke is good that is whyte and swete, and when ye droppe it on your naple, and do moue youre fynger, neyther flyeth abrode at euery sterynge,

The boke

nor wyll hange faste vpon your nayle, when ye turne it downe ward, but that whyche is betwene bothe is best.

Sometyme it chaunceth that the mylke wasteth, so that the nource can not haue sufficient to susteyne the child for ẏ whiche I wyl declare remedies leauinge out ẏ causes for brcuitie of time.

⁋Remedyes appropriate to ẏ encreasyng of mylke in the brestes.

Alneppe rootes, & fenell rootes, sodden in broth of chyckens, and afterward eaten wyth a lyttle fresch butter, maketh encrease of mylke within the brestes.

An other.

The pouder of earth wormes dryed and dronken in the brothe of a neates tonge, is a singuler experiment for the same intent.

Also the broth of an olde cocke, wyth myntes, cynamome and maces.

Ryce also sodden in cowes mylke, wyth the cromes of whyte breed, fenell seede in pouder, and a lytle sugre is exceedyng

of chyldren.

tedyng good.

¶ An other good medicyne
for the same

Take Cristall, and make it in fyne pouder, and myxe it wyth asmoche fenell seede and sugre, and vse to drynke it warme with a lytle wyne.

¶ A playster for the encrese of mylke.

Take fenelle and hoorchounde, of euery one two handfulles, anys seede foure drammes, Saffron a scruple in poudre, swete butter thre ounces, seeth them in water, and make a playster to be layed vpon the nurces brestes.

These thynges haue propertye to augment the mylke, dylle, anyse seede, fenelle, cristal, horchounde, fresh chese, honye, lettuse, beetes, myntes, carette rootes, parsneppes, the dugges or pdder of a cowe or a shepe, gootes mylke, blaunched almondes, ryce porryge, a cowes tounge dryed and made in pouder, poched egges, saffron, and the iuce of rosted veale dronken.

Thus moche of the nource, and of the

The boke

the mylke: nowe wyll I declare the infirmities of chyldren.

Althoughe (as affirmeth Plenie,) there be innumerable passions and diseases, whereu ito the bodye of man is subiecte, and as well maye chaunce in the yonge as in the olde. Yet for mooste commonlye the tender age of chyldren is chefely vexed and greued with these diseases folowynge.

Aposteme of the brayne.
Swellyng of the heed.
Scalles of the heed.
Watchyng out of measure.
Terrible dreames.
The fallyng euyll.
The palsye.
Crampe.
Styfnesse of lymmes.
Blood shotten eyes.
Watryng eyes.
Scabbynesse and ytche.
Diseases in the eares.
Nesyng out of measure.
Bredyng of teeth.

Canker

of chyldren.

Cankre in the mouth.
Quynsye, or swellyng of throte.
Coughe.
Straytnesse of wynde.
Feblenesse of the stomake & vomytyng.
Yexyng or hycket.
Colyke and rumblyng in the guttes.
Fluxe of the belly.
Stoppyng of the bellye.
Wormes.
Swellyng of the nauyll.
The stone.
Pyssyng in bedde.
Brustynge.
Fallyng of the skynne.
Chafyng of the skynne.
Small pockes and measels.
Feuers.
Swellyng of the coddes.
Sacer ignis or chingles.
Burnyng and scaldyng.
Rybbes.
Consumption.
Leanenesse.
Gogle eyes.

Of

The boke
¶ Of apostemes of the
braynes.

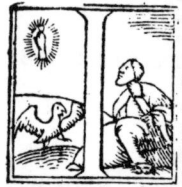

IN the fylme that couereth the brayne chaunceth oftentymes apostemation and swellyng eyther of tomoche cryinge of the chylde, or by reason of the mylke emmoderatelye hote, or excesse of heate in the blood, or of colde fleume, and is knowen by these sygnes.

Yf it be of hote matter, the heed of the chylde is vnnaturally swollē, redde, & hote in the feelynge, if it come of colde matter, it is somwhat swollen, pale, and colde in the touchyng, but in bothe cases the chylde can not reste, & is euer lothe to haue hys heed touched, cryeth and vexeth it selfe, as it were in a frenesye.

¶ Remedye.
Make a bath of mallowes, camomylle, and lyllyes sodden wyth a shepes

of chyldren.

pes heed, tyll the bones fall, and with a sponge or soft cloutes, al to bathe the heed of the chylde in a colde aposteme, wyth the brothe hote as maye be suffered, but in a hote matter wete ye brothe luke warme, or in the coolynge, and after the bath, set on a playstre, thus.

¶ A playstre

Take fenugreke, camomyll, wormwood, of euery one an handfull, seethe them in a close vessell, tyll the thyrde part be consumed, then stampe them in a mortar, and stryre them, to the which ye shall put of the same brothe agayne ynough to make a playstre, with a lytle beane floure, yolkes of egges and saffron, addyng to thē fresh butter or duckes grese suffycient, and applye it. In a colde matter lette it lye a day: but in a hote cause ye must remoue ct euery syxe houres.

¶ Of swellyng of the heed.

In

The boke

Nflation or swellynge of the heed cometh of a wyndye matter, gathered betwene the skynne and the flesh, and sometyme betwene the flesshe and the boones of the sculle, the tokens wherof are manifest ynough to the syght, by the swellynge or puffing vp, and pressed with the fynger, there remayneth a prynte, whyche is a sygne of wynde and viscous humours, ye shall heale it thus.

¶ Remedye.

Fyrst let the nourse auoyde al thinges that engendre wynde, salt or slymy humours, as beanes, peason, cles, sammon, saltfysshe, and lyke, then make a playster, to the chyldes heed, after this fashion.

Take an handefull of fenell, smallache and dylle, and seethe them in water in a close vessell, afterwarde stampe them, and wyth a lytle cumyne, and oyle of bytter almondes, make it vppe, and

of chyldren.

and laye it often to the chyldes heed, warme. In default of oyle of almons take gosegrese, adding a litle vynegre.

And it is good to bathe the place with a softe cloute, or a sponge in the broth of these herbes. Rue, tyme, maiorym, hysope, fenelle, dylle, compne, sal nitre, myntes, radysh rotes, rocket, or some of them, euer takynge heede, that there droppe no portion of the medicines iǹ ye babes eies, mouthe, or eares

⁌ Scalles of the head.

THe heades of chyldren are oftentimes vlcered, & scalled, as well when they sucke, & then moste commonlye by reason of sharpe mylke, as also when they haue bene weaned, and can go aloone. Sometymes it happeneth of an euyll complexion of humours by eatynge of rawe frute, or other euyll meates, and sometyme by longe continuynge in the sonne. manye tymes by droppynge of freshe bacon, or of salte beefe on theyr bare heedes.

Other

The boke

Other whyles they be so borne oute of theyr mothers wombe, and in all these is no greate dyfficultie tyl the heere be growen: but after that, they requyre a greater cure, and a conning hande, notwythstandynge as God shall gyue me grace, here shal be sayde remedyes for the cure of them, suche as haue ben oftentymes approued: wherein I haue entended to omytte the disputations of the dyfference of scalles, and the humours wherof they do proceade, and wyll go strayght to the composition of medicynes, folowynge the good experyence, here ensuynge.

¶ Remedyes for scalles.

Yf ye se the scalles lyke the shelles of oysters, blacke and drye, cleauynge vpon the skynne, one within an other, ye maye make a fomentation of hoote and moyste herbes, as fenugreke, holyhocke, beares breache, lyneseede, and suche other, sodden al or some of them in the brothe of netes feete, and so to bathe the sores, and after that applye
a softe

of children.

a softe playstre of the same herbes, wͭ gosegrese or butter, vsynge this styll, tyll ye se the scabbe remoued, and then wasshe it with the iuce of horehounde, smallache and betony, sodden togyther in wyne, and after the wasshynge put vpon it pouder of myrre, aloes and frākensence, or holde his heed ouer a chafyngdisshe of coles, wherin ye shall put frankensence and saunders in pouder. But yf ye se the scabbes be verye sore and mattrye wyth great payne, & burnynge of the heed,   Ye shall make an oyntment to coole tħ matter thus.

⁋ An oyntment to coole the burnynge of a sore heade.

Take whyte leade and lytarge, of euerye one, v. drammes, lye made of the asshes of a vyne, iii. drammes, oyle of roses, an ounce, waxe, an ounce, melte the waxe fyrst, than putte to the oyle & lye, wyth the resse, and in the ende, ii. yolkes of egges, make an oyntmente, & laye it to the head. This is the composition of Rasis.

An

The booke

¶ An other oyntment singuler for the same pourpose.

Take betonye, grounswel, plantayn fumytorie, and daysyes, of euery one, lyke moche, stampe them, and myngle them wyth a pounde of fresshe swynes grece, and lette them stande closed in a moyst place, viii. dayes, to putrify, thā frye them in a panne, and strayne them into a cleane vessell and ye shall haue a grene oyntmēte of a singuler operatiō for the sayde dysease, and to quenche all vnkind heates of the bodye.

Also ye muste vse to shaue the head, what so euer thiges ye doo laye vnto it

If there laketh the cleansyng of the sores, and the chylde weaned, ye shall do wel to make an oyntment of a lytle turpentyne, bulles gall, and hony and lay vpon the sores.

Also it is proued, that the vryne of a bulle, is a singuler remedy to mundifie the sores, and to lose the heares by the rootes, wythout any peyne or pille.

The iuyce also of morell, daysie lea=
ues

of chyldren.

nes and groundſwell fryed wyth greſe and made in an oyntmente, cooleth all vnkynde heates, and puſtles, of the heade.

Here is to be noted, that durynge thys dyſeaſe in a ſuckynge chylde, the nourſe muſte auoyde all ſalte, and ſower meates that engender cholere, as muſtarde, vynegre, and ſuche, and all maner frutes, (excepte a pomegranat) and ſhe muſt abſtayne in this caſe, both from egges, and frome other kynde of whyte meates in general, and aboue all ſhe maye eate no dates, figges, nor purcelane, for manye holde opynion, that purcelane hath an euylle propertye to brede ſcabbes and vlcers in the head. Moreouer the childes head may not be kepte to hote, for that is oftentymes, the cauſe of thys dyſeaſe.

Sometymes it chaunceth that there breadeth in the heade of chyldren as it were litle wartes or knobbes ſomwhat harde, and can not be reſolued by the ſayde medicines, Wherefore when ye
ſe that

The boke

ſe that none other thynge wyll healpe, yeſhal make a good oyntemente to remoue it, in maner as hereafter is declared.

❧ An excellent remedye for wartes or knobbes of the head.

Take lytarge & whyte lead, of eche a like quantitie, brymstone and quycke ſyluer quenched wyth ſpyttle of eche a leſſe quantitie, twyſe aſmoch oyle of roſes, and a ſponefulle or. ii. of vynegre, mixe them all togyther, on a marble, til they be an oyntment, and laye it on the head, & whan it hath ben drye an houre or. ii. waſſhe it of, with water, wherein was ſodden maiorym, ſaucry and mintes, vſe it thus twyſe a day, mornynge and euenynge tylle ye ſe it hole. This thyng is also good in al the other kind of ſcalles.

❧ Of watchyng out of meaſure.

Slepe is the nouryſhment and foode of a ſuckyng chylde, and aſmuch requiſyte as the very tete, wherfore whã
it is

of chyldren.

it is depryued of the naturalle reste, all the hole bodye falleth in distemper, cruditie and wekenes, it procedeth commonly by corruption of the milke, or to moche abundaunce whyche ouerladeth þe stomacke, and for lacke of good dygestion, vapoures and fumes aryse into the head, and infecte the brayne, by reason wherof the chyld can not slepe, but turneth and vexeth it selfe wyth cryeng. Therfore it shal be good to prouoke it to a naturall slepe thus, accordyng to Rasis.

Annoynte the forehead and temples of the chylde, wyth oyle of byolettes ánd vynegre, puttyng a droppe or .ii. into the nosethrylles, and yf ye can get anye syrupe of poppye, gyue it the chylde to lycke, and than make a playstre of oyle of saffron, lettuse, and the iuyce of poppie, or wet cloutes in it, and laye it ouerthwarte the temples.

Also the seades and the heades of popie, called chessbolles, stamped wyth
roses=

The booke

rosewater, and myrte wyth womans mylke, and the whyte of an egge, beaté al togyther and made in a playster, causeth the chylde to receyue hys naturall slepe.

Also an oyntmente made of the seede of popie and the heades, one ouce, oyle of lettuse, and of popie, of eche .ii. ounces, make an oyntmente and vse it.

They that can not gette these oyles, maye take the herbes, or iuyce of lettuse, purcelane, houseleke, and popie, and with womans mylke, make a playster, and laye it to the foreheade Oyle of vyolettes, of roses, of nenuphar, are good, and oyle of populeon, the broth of mallowes sodden, and the iuyce of water plantayne.

Of terryble dreames and feare in the slepe.

Oftentymes it happeneth that the chyld is afrayde in the slepe, and somtymes waketh sodaynlye, and sterteth sometime shryketh and tre-

of chyldren.

tremblethe, whyche effecte commeth of the aryſynge of ſtynkynge vapoures, oute of the ſtomacke into the fantaſye, and ſences of the brayne, as ye may perceyue by the breath of the childe wherfore it is good to gyue him a litle hony to ſwallowe, and a lytle pouder of the ſeedes of peony, and ſome tymes tryacle, in a lytle quantitie wyth mylk, and to take hede that the chylde ſlepe not wyth a full ſtomacke, but to beare it aboute wakynge, tyll parte be dygeſted and whan that it is layde, not to rocke it moche, for ouermoche ſhakynge letteth dygeſtion, and maketh the chyld manye tymes to vomyte.

☙ The fallynge euylle called in the greke tonge epilepſia.

☙.lii.   Not

The booke

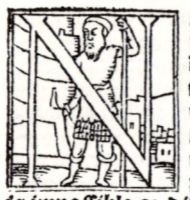

Ot only other ages but also lytle chylderne, are oftentymes afflicted, wyth thys greuous syckes, somtyme by nature recyued of the parentes, & than it is impossible, or difficile to cure, some tyme by euil & vnholsome dyete, where by there is engedred many cold & moyst humors in the brayne, wherupō this infirmitie procedeth, which if it be in one that is younge & tender, it is verye hards to be remoued, but in them ꝥ are somewhat stronge, as of. vii. yeres and vpwarde, it is more easye.

I fynde that manye thynges haue a naturall vertue agaynste the fallyng euell, not of any quality elementall, but by a singuler propertie, or rather an influence of heauen, whyche almyghtye god, hath gyuen vnto thynges here in earth, as be these and other.

Saphires, smaragdes, redde coral, pyonie,

of chyldren.

onie, mystletow of the oke taken, in the monethe of marche, and the moone decreasynge, tyme, sauein, dylle and the stone þ is foũde in the bellye of a yong swallow beyng the fyrste broode of the dame. These or one of them, hanged about the necke of the childe, saueth and preserueth it, from the sayde syckenes.
Nowe wyl I descrybe some good and holsome medicines to be taken inward for the same dysease.

If the chylde be not very young, the mawe of a leueret, dronke with water and honye, cureth the same.

¶ A medicine for the fallinge syckenes.

Take the roote of pyony, and make it into poudre and gyue it to the childe to lycke in a lytle pappe and suger.
They that are of age, maye eate of it a good quantitie atones and lykewise of the blacke seedes of the same pyonie.

¶ Item the purple violettes that creapeth on the groũde in gardeynes wyth a longe stalke, and is called in englyshe harte=

The booke

herte seace, dronken in water, or in water and honye, helpeth thys dysease in a young chylde.

Moreouer the muscle of the eke raced and gyuen in mylke, or in water & honye is good.

Also ye maye stylle a water, of the floures of lynde, it is a tree called in latyne tilia, the same wherof they make, ropes and halters of the barke, take þ same floures, and dystyll a water, and lette the pacient drynke of it nowe and than a sponefull, it is a good remedye.

℃ Item the rote of the sea thystle called Eringium in latyne, eaten in broth, or dronken is excedyng good.

℃ Some wryte that cicorie is a singuler remedye for the same dysease. It is mente by wylde cicorie, growyng in the cornes.

℃ The floures of rose marye, made in a conserua hath the same effecte in curynge this dysease.

I coulde declare many other remedies, cōmended of authours, but at thys
tyme,

of chyldren.

tyme, these shall be sufficient.

¶ Nowe I wylle entreate somewhat of the palsey.

¶ Of the palseye or shakynge of membres.

The cure of the palsey in a chyld, is not lyke to that, whyche is in elder age, for the synowes of a chylde be verye nesshe, and tender, and therfore they ought to haue a moch weaker medicyne, euermore regardynge the power of the syckenes and the vertue or debilitie of the greued paciente.

For sometymes the chylde can not lyfte nother legges, nor armes, whiche yf it happen durynge the suckyng than must the nource vse a dyet enclynyng to hote and drye, and to eate spyces, as galingale, cinamome, gynger, macis, nutmygges, and suche other, wyth rosted

and

The booke

and fryed meates, but abstayne from mylke and al maner fysshe. And it shall be good for her, to eate a lectuary made after thys sorte.

Take myntes, cynamome, cumyne, roseleaues dryed, mastyke, fenugreke, valerian, ameos doronici, zedoary, cloues, saunders, and lignum aloes, of euerye one, a dramme, muske halfe one dramme, make an electuarye wyth clarifyed honye, and let her eate of it, and gyue the chylde as much as halfe a nut euery daye to swalowe.

¶ A playster.

Take an ounce of waxe, & a dramme of euphorbium, at the potecaries, and temper it wyth oyle olyue on the fyer, and make a sereclothe, to comforte the backe bone, and the synewes.

¶ A goodly lauatory for the same pourpose.

Take lye of asshes, and seth therein baye buries, and asmoch pionie seedes, in a close vessel to the thyrde parte and wasshe the chylde often with the same

Item

of chyldren.

Item a bathe of sauerye, masorym, tyme, sage, nepte, smallage, & myntes, or some of them is very good and holesome.

Also to rubbe the backe of the chylde and the lymmes, wyth oyles of roses, and spyke, myrt togyther warme, and in stede of it ye may take oyle of bayes.

Of the crampe or spasmus.

Thys disease is often sene among chyldren and commethe verye lightlye, as of debilitye of the nerues and cordes, or els of grosse humours, that suffocate the same, the cure of the whyche is declared of authours to be done by frictions and oyntmentes that comfort the synowes and dyssolue the matter, as oyle of floure de lupce, wyth a lytle anyse, saffron and the rootes of pyonye. Item oyle of camomyl, fenugreke, and mellilote, or the herbes sodden, betonie, wormwood, vrueyne, and tyme are excedynge good to wasshe the chylde in.

Item

The booke

Item the playster of euphorbium, written in the cure of palsey.

Of the styfnes or starknes of lymmes.

Sometyme it happeneth ý the limmes are starke, and can not well come togyther, wythoute the greater peyne, whyche thynge procedeth many tymes of colde, as whā a chylde is founde in the frost or in the strete, caste awaye by a wycked mother, or by some other chaūce, although I am not ignorant that it may procede of manye other causes, as it is sayde of Rasis, and of Arnolde de villa noua, in hys booke of the cure of infantes.

And here is to be noted, a wounderfulle secrete of nature, manye tymes approued, wrytten of Auicenne in hys fyrste Canon, and of Celius Antiquarum electionum, libro. xiii. capit. xxxvi. that whan a membre is vtterly benummed and taken thorough colde, so that

the

of chyldren.

the paciente can not feele hys lymmes, nor moove them accordynge to nature, by reason of the vehement congelatiō of the blood, in suche case the chyefeste helpe or remedie is not to sette them to the fyer to receyve heate, for by that meanes, lyghtlye we se that every one swowneth, and many dye oute ryghte, but to sette the fete, legges, and armes in a payle of clere colde water, whyche immediatlye shall dissolve the congelation, & restore the bloode, to the former passage and fredome, after that ye may laye the pacient in a bedde to sweate, & gyve hym hote drynke and cawdels or a coleys of a capō hote, wyth a lytle cynamome & saffrō to cōforte þ hart. In argumēte of this cure ye maye see thus

When an apple or a pere is frosen in the wynter sette it to the fyer, and it is destroyed: but yf ye putte it into colde water it shall as well endure, as it dyd afore, whereby it doth appere that the water resolueth colde, better wyth hys moysture, than the fyer can do by reason

son of hys heate, for þ water relenteth and the fyer draweth and dryeth, as affyrmeth Galiene in his booke of elementes.

Hytherto haue I declyned by occasiō, but I truste not in vayne to the reder, nowe to my purpose.

When a yonge chylde is so takē wyth a colde, I esteme it best for to bathe the bodye in luke warme water, wherein hath ben sodden maiorym and tyme, ysope, sage, myntes, & suche other good and comfortable herbes, then to releue it wyth meates of good nouryshment, accordyng to the age and necessitie, and yf nede be, when ye se the lymmes yet to be starke, make an oyntment after this fourme.

⁋ An oyntment for styffe and stoyned lymmes.

Take a good handfull of nettles, & stampe them, then seeth them in oyle to the thyrde parte in a double vessel, kepe that oyntment in a drye place, for it wil last a great whyle, and is a singuler remedye

medye for the styfnesse that commeth of cold, and whoso anoynteth his handes and feete with it in the mornynge shall not be greued wyth colde all the daye after.

The seedes of nettles gathered in harnest & kept for ẏ same entēt, is exceding good soddē in oyle or fryed w̄ swynes grese, which thing also is very good to heale ẏ kybbes of heeles, called in latin Perniones. The vryne of a goote w̄ the donge stamped & layed to the place, resolueth the styfnesse of lymmes.

When the cause commeth not by extreme colde, but of some other affectiō of the synowes and cordes, it is best to make a bath or a fomētation of herbes that resolue and comfort the synowes, with relaxation of the grosse humours and to opē the pores as by exāple thus. Take malowes, holyhocke and dyll, of eche a handful or two, seeth them in the water of netes feete, or in broth of flesh wythout salt, wyth a handfull of bran and comyne, in the which ye shall bathe
the

of chyldren.

the chylde, as warme as he may suffre, and yf ye see necessitie, make a playstre wyth the same herbes and laye it to the griefe, wyth a lytle gosegrese, or ducckes grese, or yf it maye be gotten, oyle of camomylle, of lylyes, and of dylle. Cloutes wette in the sayde decoction, and layed about the membres, helpeth.

Of bloodshotten eyes, and other infirmities.

Omtyme þ eyes are bloodshotten and other whyles encreasynge a fylthye and whyte humoure, coueryngе the syght, the cause is often of to moche cryng, for the whiche it is good to drop in the eyes a lytle of the iuce of nyghtshade, otherwyse called morel, and to anoynt the foreheed with the same, and yf the eye swell, to wette a cloute in the iuce, and the whyte of egges, and laye it to the grefe.

If the humour be clammysshe and tough, and cleueth to the corners of the
eyes

of chyldren.

yes, so that the chylde can not open them after his slepe, it shallbe remoued with the iuce of houseleeke dropped on the eye with a fether.

When the eye is bloodshotten and redde, it is a synguler remedye to put in it, the bloode of a yonge pigion, or a doue, or a partryche, eyther hote from the byrde, or els dried and made in pouder, as subtyle as maye be possyble.

¶ A playstre for swellyng and payne of the eyes.

Take quynces and cromes of whyte bread, and seeth them in water tyl they be softe, then stampe them, and wyth a lytle saffron, and the yolkes of two egges, make a playster to the chyldes eyes and forehead. Ye maye let hym also to receyue the fume of that decoction. It is also good in the meygrym: yf ye wyl haue further, loke in the regyment of lyfe in the declaration of paynes of the heed.

¶ Of watrynge eyes.

U.i.   If

The boke

F the chyldes eyes water ouermoche wythout crying, by reason of a distillation cōmyng from the heed, Manardus teacheth a goodly playstre, to restrayne the reumes and is made thus.

Hartes horne brente to pouder, and walshed twyse, guaiacum, otherwyse called lignū sanctū, corticū thuris, antimonye, of eche one part, muske the .iii. parte of one parte, make a fyne pouder and vse it w̔ the iuce or water of fenell. These thynges haue vertue to stauche ẏ rennyng of eyes. The shelles of snayles brent, the tycke that is found in the dugges of kyne, philipendula, frankensence & the whyte of an egge layed vpō the forheed, slewort or the water wherin it is steped, tutie, the water of buddes of oke stylled, beane floure fynely syfted, and w̔ the gūme of a cherytree steped ī vinegre, & layd ouer al ẏ tēples.

⁋ Of scabbynesse and ytche.

Sometyme

of chyldren.

Ometyme by reason of excesse of heate, or sharpenesse in the mylke, throughe the nourses eatyng of salt and eygre meates, it happeneth that a chyld is sene ful of ytch by rubbing, fretyng, and chafynge of it selfe, encreasyng a scabbe called of the Grekes Psora: whyche thynge also chaunceth vnto many after they be weaned, proceding of salt & adust humoures, the cure whereof dyffereth in none other, but accordyng to ye difference of age, for in a suckyng babe ye medicines may not be so sharpe, as it maye be suffered in one that is all redye weaned. Agaynste suche vnkynde ytche, ye maye make an oyntment thus.

¶ Take water betony. ii. good handfulles, daysye leaues, and alehofe otherwyse called tunour or grounde pyne, of eche one handfull, the red docke rootes. two or thre, stampe them all togyther, and grynde them well, then myngle thẽ wyth fresshe grese, and agayne stampe

¶ The boke

them. Let them so stande .viii. dayes to putrifye tyll it be hore, then frye them out and strayne them and kepe it for ye same entent.

¶ This oyntment hath a greate effecte, both in yonge and olde, and that wythout repercussion or dryuing backe of ye matter, whyche shoulde be a peryllouse thynge for a yonge chylde.

¶ The herbe water betonye alone, is a great medicyne to quenche all vnkynde heates without daunger, or ye sethyng of it in cleare welle water, to annoynte the membres. It is a cōmon herbe, and groweth by ryuers sydes and smal renning waters, and wette places, arysing many times the heygth of a man out of the grounde, where he reioyseth, wyth a stalke foure square, and many braunches on euery syde, and also it beareth a whytysh blewe flowre very small, and in haruest it hath innumerable seedes, blacke, and as frue as the seede of tutsone or lesse, the leues bygge and long, accordyng to the grounde, full of myce,
iagged

iagged on the sydes lyke a sawe, euen as other betonye, to whome it approcheth in figure, and opteineth his name of water betonye. The sauoure of the leafe is somewhat heauye, mooste lyke to ẙ sauour of elders or walwort, but when it is brused it is more pleasaunt, whyche thyng induceth me to vary frō the myndes of them that thynke thys herbe to be Galiopsis in Dioscorides, wrytten of hym that it shoulde stynke when it is stamped, but the more thys herbe is stamped, the more swete and herbelyke it sauoureth: therfore it can not be galeopsis, and besydes that, it is neuer founde in drye and stony ground as the Galiopsis is. Neyther is thys herbe mencyoned of the newe or olde authours, as farre as I can see, but of onely Nigo, ẙ famous surgyon of our tyme in Italye, whyche wryteth on it, that thys herbe exceadeth all other in a malo mortuo (so calleth he a kynde of lepry elephantyke, or an vniuersal and sylthye scabbe of all the bodye) and in

A.iii.   lyke

The booke

lyke maner he sayeth it is good for to cure a canker in the breastes. Ye maye reade these thynges in his second boke, Capitul. iii. and hys fyfth booke of the Frenche pockes, in the thyrde chapter: where he doth descrybe thys aforesayd herbe, wyth so manyfeste tokens, that no man wyl doubt it to be water betonye, conferryng the boke and the herbe duly togyther. Moreouer he nameth in Italye a brydge where it groweth in the water in greate aboundaunce, and called of that nacyon Ilabeucratore, whych in dede the Italyons that come hyther and knowe bothe the place and the herbe do affyrme playnely, it is our water betonye,

And where as he allegeth Dioscorides in clymeno, whych by cõtemplatiõ of both hath but small affinitie or none wyth thys herbe, it was for nothynge els but lack of the tonges, which faute is not to be so hyghly rebuked in a man of his studye, applyinge hym selfe more in the practyse of surgerye, & to handye

B. iiii.   opʳatiõ

operation, wherein in dede he was nere incomparable, then he dyd to search the varyaunce of tonges, & rather regarded to declare ÿ operation of thynges ỹ truthe, then to despute vpon ÿ properties of names with eloquence.

Thus haue I declyned agayne from my matter, partly to shewe the descryptiõ of this holesome herbe, partely to satysfye the myndes of the surgions in Vigo, whiche haue hytherto redde the sayde places in vayne: & furthermore bycause there is yet none that declareth manifestly the same herbe.

⁋An other remedye for
scabbes and yche.

Take the rootes of dockes, and frye them ĩ fresh grese, then put to it a quãtitie of brymstone in pouder, and vse to rubbe the places twyse or thryse a day. Brimstone poudred and souped ĩ a rere egge healeth the scabbes, whych thyng is also very good to destroye wormes.

⁋ A goodly swete sope for
scabbes and yche.

Take

The boke

Take whyte sope halfe a pounde, & stepe it in suffycient rose water, tyl it be well soked, then take two drammes of mercurye sublymed, dissolue it in a lytle rosewater, labour the sope and the rosewater wel together, and afterward put in it a lytl: muske or cyuette, and kepe it. This sope is excedynge good to cure a greate scabbe or ytche, and that wythoute peryll, but in a chylde it shall suffyce to make it weaker of the mercurye.

¶ An other approued medicyne for scabbynesse & ytche.

Take fumpterrie, docke rootes, scabiouse, and the roote of walwort, stãpe thẽ all, & set them in freshe grese to putrifie, then frye them and strayne them in whych lycour ye shal put turpentine a lytle quantitie, brymstone, and frankensence very fynely poudred and syfted a portion, and with sufficient waxe make an oyntment on a softe fyre: thys is a syngular remedye for the same purpose. But i thys cure ye ought to gyue

the

the chylde no egges, nor anye eygre or sharpe meat, and the nurse also must auoyde the same, and not to wrappe it in to hoote, and yf neade be, to make a bath of fumiterrye, centaurye, fethersewe, tansie, wormewood, and sauge alone, yf ye se the cause of the ytche or the scabbe to be wormes in the skynne, for a bytter decoction shal destroy them and drye vp the moystures of the sores.

¶ Of diseases in the eares.

Any dyseases happē in the eares, as payne, apostemes swellynges, tynklyng and soūd i ẏ heed, stoppyng of the organes of hearynge: water, wormes, & other infortunes gotten into the eares, wherof some of them are daungerous and harde to be cured, some other expelled of nature without medicyne.

¶ Remedye for payne in the eares.

For payne in the eares withoute a manifest cause, as often chaunceth, it is a singuler remedye to take the chest wormes,

of children.

wormes, that are founde vnder barkes of trees, or in other stumpes i þ groūd and wyll tourne rounde lyke a pease, take of them a good quantytye, and seeth them in oyle, in the rynde of a pomegranade on the hote rmbres, that it brenne not, and after that strayne it and put into the eares a droppe or two luke warme, and then lette hym lye vpon the other eare, and reste. Ye maye gyue thys to all ages, but in a chylde ye must put a very lytle quantitie.

¶ An other.

The hame or skynne of an adder or a snake, that she casteth, boyled in oyle, & dropped into the eares, easeth þ payne and it is also good for an eare that matereth myngled with a lytle honye, and put in luke warme. It is also good to droppe into þ eares the iuyce of organyc and mylke.

¶ For swellyng vnder
the eares.

Paynters oyle, which is oyle of lyne seed is exedyng good for the swellyng
of

of chyldren.

of the cares, and for payne in the cares of all causes.

Item a playster made of lyneseede & oylle, with a lytle duckes grese & honye.

Yf ye se the aposteme brcke, & renne ye maye clense it with the iuce of smallache, the whyte of an egge, barly floure, & honye, which is a cōmon playstre to mundifye a sore.

When the cares haue receyued water or any other licour, it is good to take and stampe an onyon and wryng out ẏ iuce with a lytle gosegrese, and droppe it hote into the care as it may be suffred and leye hym downe one the contrarye syde an houre, after that cause hym to nese yf his age wyll suffre, wyth a lytle p̄llitorie of Spayne, or nesingpouder, and then enclyne hys care downewarde: that the water maye yssue.

¶ For wormes in the cares.

Take myrre, alocs, and the seede of colocynthis, called coloquintida of the apothecaries, a quantity of eche, seethe them ī oyle of roses, & put a litle i ẏ care

Mirre

The boke

Myrre hath a great vertue to remoue the stynche that is caused in the eares by any putrefaction, and ye better wyth oyle of bytter almons, or ye may take ye iuce of wormewood wyth hony and salt peter.

For wynde in the eares and tynklynge.

Take myrre, spykenarde, cumyne, dylle, and oyle of camomylle, and put a droppe i the eares. They that haue not all these maye take some of them, and applye it accordyng to discretion.

To amende deafnesse ye shall make an oyntment of an hares galle, and the grese or droppynge of an ele, which is a soueraypne thyng to recouer hearyng.

Of nesyng out of measure.

When a chylde neseth oute of measure, that is to saye, wt a longe continuaunce, and therby the brayne and vertues animall be febled, it is good to stoppe it, to auoyde a further i conuenience.

Whers

of chyldren.

Wherfore ye shall annoynt the heade, wyth the iuyce of purcelane, sorell, and nyghtshade, or some of them and make a playster of the whyte of an egge, and the iuyce, wyth a lytle oyle of roses, & emplayster the forheade and temples, wyth the mylke of a woman, oyle of roses, and vynegre a lytle.

If it come of colde reume, ye shall make a playster of mastyke, frankynsens, myrre, wyne, and applye it to the former parte of the head, A fume of the same receyued in flaxe, and layed vpon the chyldes head, is holsome.

Bredynge of teeth.

About ye seuenth moneth, sometyme more, sometyme lesse after ye byrthe, it is natural for a chyld for to breede teeth, in which time many one is sore vexed, wt sondrye diseases & peynes, as swelling of ye gummes & iawes, vnquiete cryenge, feuers, crampes, palsies, fluxes, reumes, & other ifirmities, speciallye whan it is longe or the teeth come forth,

forth, for the soner they apere, the better, and the more ease it is to the chylde There be diuers thynges that are good to procure an easy breedyng of teeth, among whom the chiefest is to annoynt the gummes, wyth the braynes of an hare, myxte wyth asmuch capons grece and honye, or anye of these thynges alone, is exceadynge good to supple the gummes and the synewes.

Also it is good to wasshe the chylde two or thre tymes, in a wecke, wyth warme water, of the decoction of camamyll, hollyhocke and dylle.

Fresshe butter, wyth a lyttle barlye floure, or honye, wyth the fyne pouder of frankinsence & liquirice, are commēded of good authours for ỹ same entent

And whan the peyne is greatte, and intollerable, wyth aposteme or inflammation of the goummes, it is good to make an oyntmente of oyle of roses, w the iuyce of morelle, otherwyse called nyghtshade, and in lacke of it, annoynt the iawes wythin, wyth a lytle fresshe
butter

of chyldren.

butter and honye.

For lacke of the hares brayne, ye may take the conyes, for they be also of thy kynde of hares, and called of Plinye Dasypodes, whose mawes, are of the same affecte in medicyne, or rather more, than is wrytten of authoures, of the mawes of hares.

If ye se the gummes of the chyld to aposteme or swelle wyth softe flesshe, full of matter and paynefulle, the beste shall be to annoynt the sore place wyth the brayne of an hare, & capons grece, equallye myxt togyther, and after that ye haue vsed thys, ones or twyse, annoynte the gommes, and apostematIons wyth honye.

Thyrdlye yf thys helpe not, take turpentyne myxte wyth a lytle honye in equal portion. And make a bathe for the head of the chylde, in this fourme.

Take the floures of camomylle and dyll, of eche an handeful, seeth them in a quarte of pure rennynge water, vntil they be tender, and walshe the head afore

The boke

fore anye meate, euery mornynge, for it pourgeth the superfluytye of the braynes, thorough the seames of the skull, and wythdraweth humours from the sore place, fynally comforteth ỹ brayne & all the vertues anymall of the chyld.

¶ To cause an easie bredyng of teeth, many thinges are rehersed of auctours besydes the premisses, as the fyrste cast tooth of a colte set in syluer and borne, or redde corall in lyke maner, hanged about the necke, wher vppon the chylde shulde oftentymes labour his gummes and manye other lyke, whyche I leaue out at this tyme, to auoyde tediousnes onely content to declare thys of corall, that by consent of all authours, it resisteth the force of lyghtenynge, helpeth the chyldren of the fallynge euyll, and is very good, to be made in pouder, and dronken agaynst all maner of bleedyng of the nose or fundament.

¶ Of a canker in the
    mouthe.

          Many times

of children.

Any tymes by reason of corruption of the mylke, venymous vapoures arysynge from the stomake, & of many other in fortunes, there chaueeth to brede a canker in the mouthes of chyldren, whose sygnes are manifest ynough, þ is to saye by stinkynge of the mouthe, payne in the place, contynual rennynge of spyttle, swellyng of the cheke, and when the mouth is opened agaynst the sonne, ye maye se clereye where the canker lyeth. It is so named of the latter sorte of phisitions by reason. of creppynge & eatynge forwarde & backewarde, and spreadeth it selfe abrode, lyke þ feete of a creuis, called in latyne cancer, notwithstandynge I knowe that the Greekes, and auncient latynes, gyue other names vnto this dysease, as in callyng it an vlcer, other whyles aphthe, nome, carcinomata, and lyke, whiche are al in englyshe, knowen by the name of canker in the mouthe, and although there

Æ.i.   be

The booke

be many kyndes accordyng to the matter wherof they be engendred, and therfore requyre a dyuersitie of curyng, yet for the most parte, whan they be in chylderne the cure of them all differeth verye lytle or nothyng, for the chyefe entent shall be to remoue the malignitye of the sore, and to drye vp the noysome matter and humours, than to mundify and heale, as in other kyndes of vlcers sores, and woundes.

¶ Remedies for the canker in the mouthe of children.

The drye redde roses, & violettes, of eche a lyke quantity, make them in pouder: and myxte them, with a lytle honye, thys medycyne is verye good in a tender suckynge chylde, and many tymes healeth alone, without any other thing at all. But yf ye se there be great heate & burnynge in the sore, with excedyng payne ye shal make a iuyce of purselane,

of chyldren.

selane, lettuse & nyghteshade, & wasshe the sore wyth a fyne peyce of sylke or dryue it in wyth a spoute called of the surgions a sprynge.

Thys by the grace of God, shall abate the brennynge, aswage the peyne, and kyll the venyme of the vlcer.

But yf ye se the canker yet encrease wyth greate corruption and matter, ye shal make an oyntmēt after this maner

Take myrre, galles wherewyth they make ynke, or in defaute of them, oken apples dryed, frankynsence, of eche a lyke moche, of the blake buries growynge on the bramble, taken frome the busshe whyle they be grene, the thyrde parte of al ye reste, make them al in pouder, & myxte them with asmoch honye & saffron, as is sufficient, and vse it.

¶ A stronger medicine for the canker in the mouth of children.

Take the roote of celidonie dryed, the rynde of a pomegranate, redde corall in pouder, and the pouder of a hartes horne, of eche a lyke, roche alume
       F.ii.   a lytle,

The booke

a lytle, Fyrste wasshe the place wyth wyne, or warme water, and honye, and afterwarde putte on the foresayd pouder, very fyne and subtile.

¶ In other synguler medicyne for the canker in the mouthe of all ages,

℞. ysope, sage, rue, of eche one good handefull, sethe them in wyne and water, to the thyrde part, then strayne them out, and putte in it a lytle whyte coperose, accordynge to necessytye, that is to saye, whan the sore is greatte, putte in the more, whan it is smalle ye maye take the lesse, than adde to it a quantitie of honye clarifyed, and a sponefull or. li. of good aqua vite, wasshe ye place wyth it, for it is a synguler remedy, to remooue the malyce in a shorte whyle, whyche done ye shall make a water incarnatyue and healynge thus.

℞. rybworte, betonye and daysies, of eche a handefull, sethe them in wyne, and water, and wasshe hys mouthe. ii. or. iii. tymes a day wyth the same iuce.

Moreouer

of chyldren.

Moreouer some wryte, þ cristal made in fyne pouder, hath a singuler vertue to destroye the canker, and in lyke maner the pouder of an hartes borne brēt wyth asmoche of the rynde of a pomegranade, and the iuyce of nyghtshade, is very good and holsome.

Of quinsye and swellynge of the throte.

The quisie is a daūgerous sickenes, bothe in yonge & olde, called in latyne angina, it is an inflāmation of the necke wt swellyng & great peyne, somtyme it lyeth in the verye throte, vpon the wesant pipe, & thā it is excedyng perillous for it stoppeth the breath, and straguleth the pacient anone. Other whyles it breaketh out lyke a bonche on the one syde of the necke, and than also with verye great difficultie of breathyng, but it choketh not so sone as the fyrste doeth, and it is more obedient to receyue curatiō. The signes are aparaunt to syght and besy-

The boke

des that the chylde can not crye, nether swallowe downe his meat and drynke wythout payne.

¶ Remedye.

It is good to annoynt the grefe with oyle of dylle, or oyle of camomyll, and lylies, and to laye vpon the heade, hote cloutes dipte in the waters of rosemary, lauender, and sauery.

The chyefeste remedye commended of authours in this outragious syckenes, is the pouder of a swallowe brent wyth fethers and all, and myxte wyth honye, whereof the pacient must swallowe downe a lytle, & the rest anoynted vpon the payne. They prayse also the pouder of the chyldes dunge to the chyld and of a mā to a man, brent in a potte, & anoynted with a litle honye. Somme make a compouned oyntment of bothe, the receyte is thus. ℞. of the swallowe brent, one portion: of the secōd poudre another, make it in a thycke fourme w honye, and it wyll endure longe for the same entent.

Item

of chyldren.

Item an other experimente for the quinsy and swellynge vnder the eares.

Take the mushcrim that groweth vpon an elder tre, called in englysshe Iewes eares (for it is in dede crōcled and flat, mouch lyke an eare) heate it agaist the fyer, and put it hote in any drynke, the same drynke is good and holsome for the quynsy.

Some holde opiniō that who so vseth to drynke wyth it, shall neuer be troubled wyth this dysease, and therfore carye it about with them in iorneys.

¶ Of the cough.

The cough in chyldren for the moste parte, procedeth either of a colde, or by reason of rewmes: descendynge from the head into the pypes of the longes or the breast, and that is moste commonlye by ouermoche aboundaunce of mylke, corruptynge the stomake and braync, therfore in that case, it is good to fede the childe wyth a more slendre dyete, and to an-

F.iiii. noynt

of chyldren.

noynt the heade ouer, wyth honye, and nowe and than to presse his tonge wyth your fynger, holdynge downe his head that the reumes maye issue, for by that meanes the cause of the cough shall ren out of hys mouth, & auoyde the chylde of many noughtie and slymy humours whyche done many tymes the paciente amendeth, wythout any further helpe of medicine.

For the cough in a childe.

Take gomme arabik, gumme dragagant, quynce seedes, liquyrice and penydies, at the pothecaries, breake them al togyther, and gyue the chylde to suppe a lytle at ones, wyth a draught of milk newely warme, as it cōmeth from the cowe.

Also stampe blaunched almons, and wrynge them out wyth the iuyce of fenell, or water of fenell, and gyue it to the chylde to feade wyth a lytle suger.

Agaynste the great cough, and heate in the bodye.

The heades of whyte poppye, and gumme

The booke

gumme dragagant, of eche a lyke moch longe cucumer seades, as moche as al, seth them in whaye, wyth raysons and suger, and lette the chylde drynke of it twyse or thryes a daye luke warme, or colde.

Of straytenes of wynde.

Agaynste the straytenes of brethyng whiche is no quinsie, the consent of authours do attribute a greate effecte, to lineseede made in poudre, and tempered with hony for the chylde to swallowe downe, a lytle at ones. I fynde also ẏ the milke of a mare newlye receyued of the child wyth suger, is a synguler remedye for the same pourpose.

Whyche thynge moreouer, is excedīg holsome to make the belye laxe wythout trouble.

Of weaknes of the stomacke and vomytynge.

The booke

Any times the stomacke of the chyld is so feble that it cannot retayne eyther meate or drike, in which case, and for all debilitye thereof, it is very good, to wasshe the stomake, with warme water of roses, wherin a lytle muske hath bene dyssolued for that by the odour and natural heate gyueth a comforte to all the spirituall membres.

And than it is good to roste a quynce tender, and wyth a lyttle pouder of cloues and suger, to gyue it to the chylde: to eate conserua quynces, wyth a lyttle cynamome and cloues is singuler good for the same entent. Also ye may make a iuyce of quynces & gyue it to the child to drynke wyth a lytle suger.

⁋An oyntment for the stomacke.

Take gallia muscata at the pothecaryes. xx. grayne weyght, myrrhe a very lytle, make it vp in oyntmente fourme, wyth oyle of mastyke, and water of roses sufficient, thys is a very good oynt ment

of chyldren.

ment for the stomacke.

¶ An other singuler receyte.

Take mastyk, frankinsēce, and drye redde roses, as moche as is sufficiente, make them in pouder, and temper them vp, wyth the iuyce of myntes, and a sponefull of vynegre and vse it.

¶ An other.

Take wheate floure, and parche it on a panne, tylle it begynne to brenne and waxe redde, than stampe it with vynegre, and adde to it, the yolkes of .ii. egges harde rosted, mastyke, gumme, and frankensence sufficient, make a plaistre and laye it to the stomake.

¶ To recouer an apperyte lost.

Take a good handfull of ranke and lustye rewe, and seeth it in a pynt of vinegre to the thyrde parte or lesse, and make it very stronge, wherof yf it be a childe, ye mayt take a tooste of browne bread, and stampe it with the same vynegre, and laye it playstrewyse to the stomake, and for a stronger age besydes the playstre, letts hym suppe mornynge and

The booke
and euenyng of the same vynegre.
This is also good to recouer a stomak
lost, by comynge to a fyre after a longe
iourney, and hath also a synguler ver
tue to restore a man that swowneth.

¶ An experiment often approued of Rasis for the vo-
myte of chyldren.

Rasis a solempne practicioner amõg
phisicions, affirmeth that he healed a
greate multitude of this dysease onelye
wyth the practyse folowynge which he
taketh to be of great effecte in all lyke
cases.

Fyrst he maketh as it were an electuarye of pothecarye stuffe, that is to
saye, lignum aloes, mastyke, of euerye
one halfe a dramme, galles halfe a scrupule, make a lectuarye wyth syrupe of
roses, and gallia muscata and sugre.

Of this he gaue the children to eate a
very lytle at ones and oftē. Afterward
he made a playster thus. ℞, mastyke, a
loes, sloes, galles, frankensence, and
brent bread, of eche a like portion, make
a plai-

of chyldren.

a plaistre with oyle and syrupe of rose to be layed to the childes stomake hote.

⁋An other oyntment for the stomake, descrybed of Wilhel. Placentino.

Take oyle of mastyke or of wormewood .ii. ounces, waxe, thre ounces, cloues, maces, and cynamome of eche, thre drammes, make an oyntment, addynge in the ende a lytle vynegre.

The yolke of an egge harde rosted, mastyke, frankensence and gumme, made in a plaistre with oyle of quinces, is exredyng good for the same purpose.

⁋Of ycarynge or hycket.

It chaunceth oftentymes that a chylde yexeth out of measure. Wherfore it is expedyent to make the stomake eygre afore it be fed, & not to replenysshe it wyth to moche at ones, for this disease commonly procedeth of fulnes: for yf it come of emptinesse, or of sharpe humours in the mouth of the stomake, whiche is
seldom

The booke

seldom sene: the cure is thē very diffycil and daungerous.

¶ Remedye.

When it cōmeth of fulnesse ẏ a child yexeth incessauntlye without measure and that by a lōg custome, it is good to make hī vōmyt w a fether, or by some other light meanes, ẏ the matter which causeth the yexynge, maye yssue and vncombre the stomak, that done, bryng it a slepe, and vse to annoynt ẏ stomak wyth oyles of castor, spyke, camomyll, and dyll, or two or thre of them, ioyned togyther warme.

¶ Of colycke and rumblynge in the guttes.

Peyne in the belly is a cōmon dysease of children, it cōmeth eyther of woormes, or of takinge colde, or of euyll mylke, the sygnes thereof are to well knowen for the childe can not rest, but cryeth, ⁊ fretteth it self, ⁊ manye tymes, can not make theyr vryne, by reason of wynde,

of chyldren.

wynde, that oppresseth the necke of the bladder, & is knowen also, by the mēbre in a man child, whyche in this case, is alwaye styffe, & pryckynge, moreouer ỹ noyse & roblyng in the guttes, hyther & thither declareth ỹ child to be greued, with wynde in the bellye and colik.

¶ Cure.

The nourse muste auoyde all maner meates that engēdre winde, as beanes, peason, butter, harde egges, and suche.

Then wasshe the chyldes bellye wyth hote water wherin hath ben sodden comyne, dylle and fenell, after that make a playstre of oyle and waxe, and clappe it hote vpon a cloth vnto the bellye.

¶ An other good playstre for the same entent.

Take good stale ale and fresh butter, seeth them with an handfull of comyne poudred, and after put it all togyther into a swynes bladder, & bynde the mouthe faste, that the lycoure yssue not out, thē wynde it in a cloth, & turne it vp and downe vpō the belly as hote

as the

The booke

as the pacient maye suffer, this is good for the colyke after a sodayne colde, in all ages, but in chyldren ye must beware ye applye it not to hote.

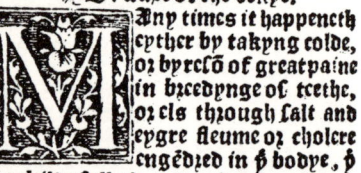

¶ Of fluxe of the bellye.

Any times it happeneth eyther by takyng colde, or by reson of great paine in breedynge of teethe, or els through salt and eygre fleume or cholere engedred in ye bodye, ye childe falleth into a sodayne laxe, which yf it longe continue & be not holpen, it may bryng ye pacient to extreme leanesse, & consumption: wherfore it shal be good to seke some holsome remedy & to stoppe the rennyng of the fluxe thus.

¶ Remedye for the fluxe in a chylde.

Fyrst make a bath of herbes that do restrayne, as of plantayne, saint Johns weede called ypericon, knotgrasse, bursa pastoris and other suche, or some of them, and vse to bath him in it as hote as he may wel suffre, then wrappe him
in with

of children.

in hi clothes, & laye him downe to slepe.

And yf ye se by this twyse or thryse vsynge, that the belye be not stopped: Ye maye take an egges yolke harde rosted, and grynde it with a lytle saffron, myrrhe and wyne, make a playster, and applye it to the naupl hote. Yf this suc cede not, then it shalbe necessarye for to make a poudre to gyue him in his meate with a litle sugre and in a smal quantitie thus.

Take the poudre of hartes horne bret, ẏ poudre of gootes clawes, or of swynes clawes bret, the poudre of the seede of roses whyche remayne in the berye when the rose is fallen, of euerye one a portion, make them very fine, & with good redde wyne or almon mylke, and wheat floure, make it as it were a paste and drye it in lytle balles tyll ye se necessitie, it is a singuler remedie in al suche cases.

Item the mylke wherin hath bene sodden whyte paper, and afterwarde quenched, manye hote yrons or gaddes

The booke

of stele, is excedynge good for the same
entent to drynke.

And here is to be noted, that a natural flure is neuer to be feared afore the
.vii. day, and except there issue blood,
it ought not to be stopped afore the
sayde tyme.

Pouder of the herbe called knotgrasse or the iuce therof in a posset dronken, or a playstre of the same herbe, &
of bursa pastoris, bolearmenye, and the
iuce of plantayne with a lytle vynegre,
and wheate flour is excedynge good
for the same cause.

Also the rynole mawe of a yonge suckynge kydde gyuen to the chylde, the
weight of .x. graynes, with ye yolke of
an egge softe rosted, and let the patient
abstayne from mylke by the space of .ii.
houres before and after, in stede wherof ye may gyue a rosted quince or a warden wyth a lytle sugre and cynamome
to eate.

¶ Item an other goodly recepte
for the same entent,

Take

of chyldren.

Take sorel seed and the kernelles of greate raysyns dryed, ackorne cuppes, and the seed of whyte poppe: of eche. ii. drames, saffron a good quantitie, make them in pouder and tempre them wyth the iuce of quynces, or syrupe of red roses this is a soueraynge thyng in al fluxes of the woumbe.

Many other thynges are wrytten of authours in the sayd discase, whiche I here leaue out for breuitie: and also bycause the afore reherced medicynes are suffycient ynough in a case curable: yet wyll I not omytte a goodly practyse in the sayde cure. The pesyll of an hart or a stagge dryed in pouder and dronken, is of great and wonderful effect in stoppyng a fluxe. Whiche thyng also is approued in the lyuer of a beaste called in Englysshe an otter. The stones of him dronken in pouder, a lytle at ones thryty daies togyther, hath healed men for euer of the fallyng euyll.

⁜ Of stoppynge of the bellye.

Fa.ii.   Euen

The boke

Uen as a fluxe is daungerous, so is stoppynge and hardenesse of ye belly greuous & noysome to the chylde, and is often cause of the colycke and other diseases.

Wherfore in this case ye muste alwaye put a lyttle hony into ye chyldes meate and lette the nource gyue hym honye to sucke vpon her fynger, and yf this wyl not helpe, then the nexte is to myxe a lytle fyne and cleare turpentyne, wyth honye, and so to resolue it in a saucer, and let the chylde suppe of it a lytle.

This medicine is descrybed of Paulus Agineta, and receyued of dyuers other as a thyng very holsome and agreinge to the nature of the chylde, for it doeth not only losen ye belly without grefe or daunger, but doth also purge the lyuer and the longes, with the splene and kidneyes generally comforting all the spirituall membres of the bodye,

The gall of an oxe or a cowe layed
vpon

of chyldren.

vpon a cloute on the nauylle, causeth a chylde to be loose bellyed, lykewyse an emplaystre of a rosted onyon, the galle of an oxe, and butter layed vpon the belye as hote as he maye suffre. Yf these wyll not helpe, ye shal take a lytle cotten, and rolle it, and dypped in the sayde gall, put it in the fundament.

¶ Of wormes.

Here be dyuerse kyndes of wormes in ye bellye, as longe, shorte, rounde, flat and some smalle as lyce, they be all engendred of a crude, grosse, or phlegmatyke matter, and neuer of choler nor of melancholy, for all bytter thynges kylleth them, and al swete meates that engendre fleume, nouryssheth and feedeth the same. The signes dyffer accordyng to the wormes. For in the long & round the pacient comonly hath a drye cough, payne in the belly about ye guttes, some tyme crayinge & treblyng in ye night, & starte sodaynely, & fall aslepe agayne.

Ja.iii. others

The booke

other whyles they gnasshe and grynde theyr teeth togyther, the eyes waxe holowe, with an eygre loke, & haue greate delyte in slombryng, and sylence, verye loth when they are a waked. The pulse is incertayne, and neuer at one staye, sometyme a feuer with greate colde in the ioyntes, which endureth thre or .iiii. houres i the nyght or daye, many haue but small desire to meate, and when they desyre, they eate verye greedelye, whych yf they lacke at theyr appetyte, they forsake it a great whyle after, the hole body consumeth and wareth leane the face pale or blewe: somtyme a fluxe somtymes vomyte, and in some the belye is swollen as styffe as a taberet.

The longe and brode wormes are knowen by these sygnes, that is to saye, by yelownesse or whyttishnesse of the eyes intollerable hungre, greate gnawyng and gryppyng in the bellye, specyally afore meat, water commyng oute at the mouth, or at the foundament, continuall ytche and rubbyng of the nosethrylles,

sonken

of chyldren.

sonken eyes and a stynkyng breath, also when the person doth his easement, there appeareth in the donge lytle flat substaunces, moche lyke the seedes of cucumers or gourdes.

⁋The other lesse sorte are engendred in the great gutte, and may wel be knowen by the exceedynge ytche in the fundament within, and are ofttymes sene commyng out with the excrementes.

⁋They be called of phisions ascarydes

⁋Remedy for wormes
in chyldren.

⁋The herbe that is founde growyng vpon oysters by the sees syde, is a synguler remedye to destroye wormes, and is called therfore of the Grekes Scolytabotani, that is to saye, the herbe that kylleth wormes: it must be made in pouder, and gyuen wyth sweate mylke to the chylde to drynke. The Phisicions call the same herbe coralino.

⁋A singuler receyte for
to kyll wormes.
⁋Take the gall of a bull or oxe, new-
lye-

lye kylled, and stampe in it an handfull of good comyne, make a playstre of it, & lay it ouer all the bellye, remouyng the same euery syxe houres.

Item the galle of a bulle wyth seedes of colocynthis called colloquintida of the pothecaryes, and an handfulle of baye beryes well made togyther in a playstre, with a sponefull of strong vinegre, is of greate effecte i̅ y̅ same case.

Yf the chylde be of age or stronge complexion, ye may make a fewe pilles of aloes, and the pouder of wormeseed, then wynde them in a pece of a syngyng lofe, and annoynt them ouer wyth a lytle butter: and lette them be swalowed downe hole without chewyng.

¶ Of swellyng of the nauill.

In a chylde lately borne, and tender, sometyme by cuttyng of the nauyll to nere, or at an inconuenient season, sometyme by swadlynge or byndynge anysse, or of moche cryng, or coughynge, it happeneth otherwhyles, that

of chyldren.

that the nauyll aryseth and swelleth wyth greate payne and apostemation, the remedy wherof is not muche differente from the cure of vlcers, sauynge in thys that ye ought to applye thynges of lesse attraction, then in other kynde of vlcers, as for an example, ye maye make an oyntment vnder thys fourme. Take spyke or lauender halfe an ounce, make it in poudre, and wyth thre ounces of fyne and cleare turpentyne, tempre it in an oyntment, addyng a portion of oyle of swete almons. But yf it come of crynge, take a lytle beane floure: and the asshes of fyne lynnen cloutes brent, and tempre it with redde wyne and honye, and laye it to the sore.

¶ A playstre for swellyng in the nauill.

Take cowes donge, and drye it in poudre, barlye floure, and beane floure of eche a porcyon, the iuyce of knotgrasse a good quantitie, compne a lytle, make a playster of all and set it to the nauyll.

In

The booke
¶ An other.

Take cowes donge and seeth it in the mylke of the same cowe, and laye it on the grefe, This is also marueylouse effectuall to helpe a soddayne ache, or swellyng in the legges.

¶ Of the stone in chyldren.

The tender age of chyldren as I sayd afore, is vexed and afflycted with manye greuous and peryllous diseases, amonge whome there is few or none so violent or more to be feared in them, then that whyche is mooste feared in all kynde of ages, that is to saye ye stone, an houge and a pityfull disease, euer the more encreasyng in dayes, the more rebelling to the cure of Physycke.

Therfore is it excedyng daungerouse whan it falleth in chyldren, for asmoch as neyther the bodyes of them may be well purged of the matter antecedent called humor peccans, nor yet can abide any vyolent medecyne hauynge power
to breake

of chyldren.

to breake it, by reason wherof the sayed dysease acquyreth suche a strengthe aboue nature, that in processe of tyme it is vtterlye incurable.

Yet in the begynnyng it is oftentymes healed thus

Fyrste lette the nurse be wel dyeted or the chylde, yf it be of age, abstayning from all grosse meates, and harde of digestion, as is beafe, bacon, saltemeates and cheese, than make a pouder of the roote of peonye dryed, and myngle it wyth asmoche honye as shal be suffycient, or yf the child abhorre hony, make it vp wyth suger molten a lytle vppon the cooles, and gyue thereof vnto the chylde, more or lesse, accordynge to the strengthe, twyse a daye, tyll ye se the brync passe caselye, ye maye also gyue it in a rere egge, for wythout dout it is a syngulcr remedye in chyldren.

⁋ An oyntment for the same.

Oyle of scorpions, yf it may be gotten, is exceding good to annoynt wyth all the membres, and the nether parte

of

The boke

of the bellye, ryghte agaynste the bladder, ye may haue it at the pothecaries.

¶ A singuler bathe for the same entent.

Take mallowes, holyhock, lylie rotes, lynseed, and parietarye of the wal, seeth them all in the brothe of a shepes head, and therein vse to bathe the chyld oftentymes, for it shal open the strayt nes of the condytes, that the stone may issue, swage the payne, and brynge oute the grauell with the vryne, but in more effecte whan a playster is made, as shal be sayde hereafter, and layed vpon the raynes, and the bellye, immediatly after the bathynge.

¶ A playster for the stone.

Take parietarie of the wall, one portion, & stampe it, doues dounge an other portion, and grynde it, that frye them bothe ī a panne, wyth a good quan titye of fresshe buttyre, and as hote, as may be suffered, laye it to the belly and the backe, and from iiii. houres. to. iiii. let it be renewed.

Thys

of chyldzen.

This is a soueraygne medicine in all maner ages.

Item an other pouder whiche is made thus

Take the kernels or stones that are founde in the frupte, called openers or mespiles, oz of some, medlars.

Make them in fyne pouder, whiche is wounderfull good for to breake the stone wythout daunger, bothe in yong and olde.

The chestwoormes dryed and made in fyne pouder, taken wyth the brothe of a chicken, oz a lyttle suger, helpeth them, that can not make theyz vryne.

Of pyssynge in the bedde.

Anytimes for debilitye of vertue retentiue of the reynes oz bladder as wel olde men as children are oftentymes annoyed, whan their vrī issueth out either ī theyz sleepe oz wakyng agaynst theyz willes, hauyng no power to reteyne it whā it cōmeth, therefoze yf they wil be holpe, fyrst they must auoyde all fatmeates, til

the

The booke

the vertue retentiue be restored agayne and to vse thys pouder in theyr meates and drynkes.

Take the wesande of a cocke, & plucke it, than brenne it in pouder, and vse of it twise or thryes a daye. The stones of an hedgehogge poudred is of the same vertue.

Item the clawes of a goate, made in pouder dronken, or eaten in pottage.

If the paciente be of age, it is good to make fyne plates of leade, wyth holes in them, and lette them lye often to the naked backe.

Of brustynge.

The causes of it in a childe are many, for it maye come of very lyghte occasions, as of great cryeng, & stoppynge the breath byndynge to strayte, or by a falle, or of to greate rockynge, & suche lyke, maye cause the filme that spreadeth ouer the ballye, to breake or to slacke, and so the guttes fall downe, into the cod, whych yf it be not vtterly vncurable, maye be
healed

of chyldren.

healed after thys sorte.

¶Fyrste laye the pacient so vpon his backe, that hys heade maye be lower than his heales, than take and reduce the bowels wyth youre hande, into the due place, afterwarde ye shall make a playster to be layde vppon the coddes, and bounde wyth a lace rounde aboute the backe, after thys fourme.

¶Take rosyn, frankynsence, mastyke, compne, lynesseed, and anyse seed of euerye one a lyke, pouder of osmonde rootes, that is to saye, of the brode ferne, the iiii. parte of all, make a playster w sufficient oyle olyue, and fresshe swynes grece, and sprede it on a lether, and let it continue (except a great necessity) two or three weekes, after that applye an other lyke, tylle ye see amendment. In this case it is verye good to make a poudre of the heares of an hare, & to temper it with suger or conserua roses and gyue it to the chylde twyes euery day.

¶If it be aboue the age of vii. yere, ye

maye

maye make a singuler recepte in drink to be taken euerye daye twyse, thus.

¶ A drynke for one that is brosten.

Take matfelon, daysies, comferye and osmūdes, of euery one a lyke, seeth them in the water of a smythes forge, to ye thyrde parte, in a vessel couered, on a softe fyer, than strayne it and giue to drynke of it, a good draughte at ones, mornynge and euenyng, addynge euermore in his meates, and drynkes, the pouder of the heare of an hare, beynge dryed,

¶ Of fallynge of the fundamente.

Any tymes it happeneth that the gutte called of the latynes rectum intestinū, falleth out, at the fundament, and can not be gotten in agayne wythout peyne and laboure, whyche dyscase is a common thynge in children, commyng oftentymes of a sodayne colde or a lōge laxe, and may wel be cured by these subscribed medicines.

It

of chyldren.

If the gutte hath ben longe out, and be so swollen that it cānot be reposed, or by coldenes of the ayre be congeled, the best counsell is to let the chylde syt on a hote bathe, made of the decoction of mallowes, hollyhocke, lyneseed, and the rootes of lyllies, wherein ye shall bathe the foundamente, wyth a softe cloute or a sponge, and whan the place is suppled thruste it in agayne, whyche done, than make a pouder thus.

A pouder for fallynge of the foundament.

Take the poudre of an hartes horne brent, the cuppes of acornes dryed, rose leaues dryed, goates clawes brent, the rynde of a pomegranate, and of galles, of euerye one, a portion. Make them in pouder, and strowe it on the fundament. It shall be the better, yf ye put a lytle on the gutte, afore it be reposed in ý place, & after it be setled, to put more of it vpon the fundamēt, than binde it in with hote lynnen clothes, and gyue the chylde quynces, or a rosted warden

The booke
to eate wyth cinamome and suger.
¶ An other good pouder
for the same.

Take galles, myrre, frankynsence, mastyke, and aloes, of euery one a lytle make thē in a pouder, and strawe it on the place.

A lytle tarre wyth gosegrece is also verye good in this case.
¶ An other good remedye.

Take the wolle frome betwene the legges, or of the necke of a shepe, which is full of sweate and fattie, than make a iuyce of vnsette leekes, and dippe the wolle in it, and laye it to the place as whotte, as maye be suffered, and whan it waxeth colde remoue it and apply an other hote, this is a very good remedy for fallynge of the fundament.

If the chylde prouoke many tymes to seege, and can expell nothynge, that dysease is called of the Grekes tenes=mos, for the whyche it shall be verye good to applye a playster made of gar=deyne cressys & comyncin, lyke quanti=
tye

The booke

tye, frye them in butter, and laye it on the bellye as hote as he maye suffre.

It is also cōmended, to fume the nether partes wyth turpentyne & pitche, & to sytte longe vpon a bourde of cedre, or iunyper, as hote as maye be possible.

⁋ Chafynge of the skynne.

IN the flanckes, armeholes, & vnder the eares, it chaunceth often tymes ẏ the skyn fretteth, either by the childes own vryne, or for the defaut of wasshig or elles by wrappynge and keppynge to hote.

Therfore in the begynnynge, ye shal annoint the places, with fresshe capons grece, then yf it wylle not heale, make an oyntment, and laye it on the place.

⁋ An oyntement for chafyng
and gallynge.

Take the roote of the floure deluyce dryed, of redde roses dryed, galingale and mastycke, of eche a lyke quantitye, beate them in to moste subtyle pouder: than wyth oyle of roses, or of lynseed make a softe oyntment.

Bb, ii.   Item

The booke

Item the lounges of a wether dryed, and made in very fyne pouder, healeth all chafynges of the skine, and in like maner the fragmentes of shomakers lether, brent and caste vpon the place, in as fyne pouder as is possyble, hath the same affecte, whych thyng is also good for the gallynge or chafynge of the fete of what so euer cause it conuneth.

Item beanfloure, barlye floure, and the floure of fytches tempered wyth a lytle oyle of roses, maketh a souerayne oyntment for the same entent.

If ye chafynges be great, it is good to make a bathe of holyhocke, dyl, violets & lineseed w a lytle bra, than to wasshe the same places oftentymes, and laye vpon the sore, some of ye same thinges.

The decoction of plantayne, bursa pastoris, horsetayle and knotgrasse, is excedynge good to heale all chafynges of the skynne.

¶ Of smal pockes & measylles.

This dysease is common and famililier called of the grekes by the generall

of chyldren.

call name of exanthemata, and of Plinie, papule et pituite eruptiones, not wythstandyng the consent of wryters, hath obteyned a destinction of it, in.ii. kyndes, that is to saye variol i the measyls, and morbilli called of vs the small pockes.

¶They be bothe of one nature, & procede of one cause, sauynge that the mesyls are engendred, of the instamation of blood, and the smal pockes of the instammation of bloode myngled wyth choler.

¶The signes of them bothe, are so manifest, to syghte, that they nede no farther declaration, for at the fyrste some haue an ytche and a fretyng of the shyn as yf it had ben rubbed wyth nettles, payne in the head and in the backe, the face redde in coloure and flecked, feare in the slepe, great thyrste, rednes of the eyes, beatynge in the temples, shotyng and pryckyng thorough all the bodye, then anone after, when they breake out they be sene of dyuers faschyons, & four mes,

mes, somtyme as it were a drye scabbe
or a leprye spreading ouer al the mēbres
other whiles i pusshes, piples, & wheles,
rennyng with moch corruption & matter, & with greate peyne of the face and
throte, dryenesse of the tōge, horcenes
of voyce, and in some quiueryngs of
the harte, with swownyngs.

ℂ The causes of these euel affections,
are rehersed of authours, to be chyefly
foure.

Fyrste of the superfluyties whyche
myght be corrupte in the woumbe of ye
mother, the chylde there beyng, and re=
ceyuynge the same into the poores, the
whyche at that tyme for debility of nature, coulde not be expelled, but ye child
increasynge afterwarde in strengthe,
be dryuen oute of the veynes, into the
vpper skynne.

Secondarilie it maye come of a corrupte generation, that is to saye whan
it was engendred in an euyl season, the
mother beynge syke of her natural in-
firmitye, for suche as are begotten that
tyme

tyme verye seldome escaye the disease of lepiye.

The thyrde cause maye be an euyll dyete of the nourse, or of the chylde it selfe, whan they feade vppon meates, that encrease rotten humours, as milk and fyshe both at one meale, lykewise excesse of eatynge and drynkynge, and surfeyte.

Fourthlye this dysease commeth by the waye of contagion, whan a sycke person infecteth an other, and in that case it hath great affinitie wyth the pestylence. ¶Remedye.

The best and most sure helpe in this case, is not to meddle wyth any kynde of medicines, but to let nature woorke her operation, not wythstandynge yf they be so slowe in commynge oute, it shall be good for you to gyue the chyld to drinke, sodden mylke and saffron, & so kepe hym close and warme whereby they maye the soner issue forthe, but in no case to administre anye thynge that might eyther represse the swellynge of

The booke

the skynne or to coole the heate that is wythin the membres. For yf thys dysease which shuld be expelled by a natural action of the body to the long heal the afterwarde of the pacient, were by force of medicine cowched in agayne, it were euen ynough to destroye þ chyld. ¶Therfore abide the ful breaking out of þ saide wheales, & then (yf they be not ripe) ease þ chyldes peyne by makynge a bath of holihock, dil, camomil & fenel, yf they be rype & mater, then take fenell wormewood and sage, and seeth them in water, to the thyrde part, wher in ye maye bathe him with a fyne cloth or a spōge. Alwayes prouyded þ he take no colde durynge þ tyme of his syckenesse.

¶The wyne wherin fygges haue ben sodde is singuler good in þ same case, & may be well vsed in all tymes & causes.

¶Yf the wheles be outragyous and great, with moche corrosiō and venim some make a decoction of roses and plātayne, in the water of oke, and dissolue in it a lytle englysh honye and cāphore.

¶The

of chyldren.

¶The decoction of water betonye, is approued good in the sayde dyseases. Likewyse the oyntmēt of herbes, wher of I made mention in the cure of scabbes, is excedynge holsome after the sores are rype.

Moreouer it is good to droppe in y̌ pacientes eyes .v. or vi. tymes a daye a lytle rose or fenel water, to comforte the syght, lest it be hurte by contynuall rennig of matter. This water must be mynistred in the somer colde, and in the winter ye ought to aply it luke warme

The same rose water is also good to gargle in his mouthe, yf the chylde be then payned in the throte.

And lest the condites of the nose shuld be stopped, it shall be very expedient to let hym smell often to a sponge wete in the iuce of sauerye, stronge vynegre, & a lytle rosewater.

¶To take awaye the spottes & scarres of the smal pockes and measels.

¶The blood of a bulle or of an hare is moche cōmēded of authours to be an
nointed

The booke

noynted hote vpon the scarres, and also the lycour that yssueth out of shepes clawes, or gootes clawes hette in the fyre. Item the drypppyng of a cygnet or swanne layed vpon the places oftentymes hote.

¶ Feuers.

YF the feuer vse to take ỹ chylde with a great shakyng, and afterwarde hote, whether it be cottidian or tercian, it shal be singuler good to gyue it in drynke, the blacke seedes of Peonye made in fyne pouder, searced and myngled with a lytle sugre.

Also take plátayne, fetherfew and veruepn, and bathe the chylde in it ones or twyse a daye, bynding to the pulces of the hādes and feet a playstre of ỹ same herbes stamped, and prouoke the childe to sweate afore the fytte commeth.

Some gyue counsell in a hote feuer, to applye a colde playstre to the brest, made in this wyse. Take the iuyce of wormewood, plátayne, mallowes and houselceke, and temper in thē asmoch barlye floure as shal be suffycyent, and vse it.

of chyldren.

vse it. Or thus, and more better in a weake pacyent.

Take drye roses and poudre them then tempre the poudre wyth the iuyce of endyue or purcelane, rose water, and barlye floure, and make a playstre to the stomake.

Item an oyntment for his temples armes and legges, made of oyle of roses, and populeon, of eche lyke moche.

A good medicine for the ague in chyldren.

Take plantayne with the roote, and wash it, then seeth it in fayre runnynge water to the thyrde parte: whereof ye shall gyue it a draughte (yf it be of age to drynke) with sufficient sugre, & laye the sodden herbes as hoote as maye be suffred, to the pulses of the handes and feet. This must be done a litle afore the fytte, and afterward couer it wt clothes

The oyle of nettles wherof I spake in the title of styfnesse of lymmes, is exceedynge good to annoynt the membres in a colde shakynge ague.

Of

The boke

¶ Of swellynge of the coddes.

To remoue the swellynge of the coddes, proceedynge of ventositie, or of any other cause (excepte brustynge,) whether it be with inflammation or without, here shall be rehersed manye good remedyes, of whyche ye maye vse, accordyng to the qualitye and quantitye of the grefe: alway prouided that in this disease, ye maye i no case applye any repercussyues, that is to saye, set no colde herbes to dryue the matter backe, for it would than returne agayne into the body, and the congelation of such a sinowye mēbre, would peraduenture mortifye the hole. And aboue all, ye maye set no plaster to the stones, wherin humlocke entreth, for it wyll depryue them for euer of theyr growynge, and not only them but the brestes of wenches, whan they be annoynted therewyth, by a certeyne qualitye, or rather an euyl property beinge in it.

¶ A goodly playster for swellyng
of the

of children.

of the stones.

Take a quarte of good ale worte and set it on the fyre to seethe wyth the cromes of browne bread strongly leuened, and a handefull of comyne or more in pouder, make a playster wyth all thys and sufficiente beane floure, and apply it to the grefe, as hote as may be suffered. ¶ In other.

Take cowes donge, and seethe it in mylke, than make a playster, and laye it metelye hote vpon the swellynge.
¶ In other.

Take comyne, anyseseed, and fenugreke, of eche a like portion, seeth them in ale and stampe them, then tēpre them with fresh maye butter, or a lytle oyle olyue, and applye it to the sore.
¶ In other

Take camomyll, holyhocke, lynseed and fenugreke, seethe them in water, & grynde all togyther, then make a playster wyth an handfull of beane floure, and vse it.
¶ In other in the begynnyng

of the

The booke
of the griefe.

Yf there be moche inflammation or heate in the coddes, ye maye make an oyntment of plantayne, the whyte and yolke of an egge, and a portion of oyle of roses, styrre them well aboute, & applye it to ye grefe twyse or thryse a day.

When the payne is intollerable, and the chylde of age, or of stronge complexion yf the premisses wyll not helpe, ye shall make a playstre after this sorte. Take henbane leaues, an handful and an halfe, mallowe leaues, an handfull, seeth them well in cleare water, then stampe them and styrre them, and with a lytle of the broth, beane floure, barly floure, oyle of roses and camomyll suffycient, make it vp and set on ye swellyng luke warme. Henbane as Auicēne sayth, is excedynge good to resolue the hardnesse of the stones by a secret qualitie. Notwithstandynge, yf it come of wynde, it shalbe better to vse the sayde playsters ye are made with compne, for that is of a singuler operatiō in dissol-

uyng

Of sacer ignis or chingles.

IN Greke herisipelas, and of the Latines Sacer ignis, our Englysshe women call it the fyre of Saynt Anthonye, or chingles, it is an inflammatiō of membres with excedyng burnynge and rednesse, harde in the feelynge, and for the most parte crepeth aboue the skynne or but a lytle depe within the flesshe.

It is a greuous payne, and maye be lykened to the fyre in consumyng. Wherfore the remedyes þ are good for burning are also very holsome here in this case. And fyrste the greene oyntment of herbes described in þ chapter of ytche, is of good effect also in this cure, moreouer the medicines þ are here described

Take at the pothecaries of vnguētū Galeni an ounce and an halfe, oyle of roses two ounces, vnguenti popalcon one ounce, the iuce of plātayne, nightshade one ounce or more, the whites of
the

The booke

thre egges, heate them altogyther, & ye shal haue a good oyntmēt for the same purpose. ¶ An other.

Take earthwormes and stāpe them in vynegre, then annoynt the grefe euery two houres.

Itē the dōge of a swanne, or in lacke of it the donge of a gose stamped w̄ the whyte and yolke of an egge, is good.

Itē doues donge stāped in salet oyle or other, is a singuler remedye for the same purpose.

¶ Of burnyng and scaldyng.

For burnyng & scaldyng whether it be w̄ fier, water, oyle lead, pytche, lyme, or any such infortune: ye must beware ye set no repercussiue at þ fyrst, that is to saye, no medicine of extreme colde, for that myght chaunce to dryue the feruēt heate into the synowes & so stoppe the poores, that it coulde not issue: whereof shulde happen moche inconuenience in a great burning (but in small it coulde not be so daungerous,) wherfore þ best
is when

is when ye se a membre eyther brent or scalded, as is sayde afore.

Take a good quantitie of bryne, which is made of water and salt, not to exceadynge eygre or stronge, but of a meane sharpenesse: and with a clout or a spōge bathe the membre in it colde, or at the leest bloodwarme, thre or foure houres togyther, the longer the better: For it shall aswage moche of the peyne, open the pores, cause also the fyre to vapour and gyue a great comfort to the weake membre. Then annoynt the place with one of these medicynes.

Take oyle of roses one part, swete creme two partes, honye halfe a parte, make an oyntment and vse it.

Item all the medicines descrybed in the last chapiter, are of great effecte in this case, lykewyse the grene oyntment made of water betonye.

Item a soueraypne medicyne for burnynge and scaldynge, and all vnkynde heates is thus made. Take a dosen or more of harde rosted egges, and put the

The booke

yolkes in a pot on the fyre by themselfe, without lycour, styrre them and braye them with a stronge hande, tyl there aryse as it were a froth or spume of oyle to the mouthe of the vessell, then presse the yolkes and reserue the lycour, this is called oyle of egges: a very precyous thyng in the forsayde cure.

Moreouer there is an oyntment made of shepes dõg fryed in oyle or in swines grece, thã put to it a lytle waxe, & vse it

Also take quycke lyme and wasshe it in veriuce, ix. or x. tymes, than mingle it w[ith] oyle, & kepe it for the same entent.

Item the iuce of the leaues of lillies v. partes, and vyneegre one part, honye a lytle, maketh an excellent medicine, not onelye for this entent, but for all other kynde of hote and rennyng vlcers. ¶ Note that what so euer ye vse in this case, it must be laide vnto, blood warme. Also for auoydyng of a scarre, kepe the sore alwaye moyst with medicyne,

¶ Of kybes

Th[e]

of chyldren.

The kybes of ye heeles, are called in latyn perniones, they procede of colde, & are healed w^t these subscrybed remedies. A rape rote, rosted w^t a litle fresh butter is good for the same grefe.

Item a dosen fygges, sodden & stamped wyth a lytle goose grece, is good.

Earthe wormes sodden in oyle, hath the same effecte.

Item ye skynne of a mouse clapped al hote vpon the kybe, wyth the heare outwarde, and it shulde not be remoued durynge .iii. dayes.

¶ A playster for a kybed heele.

Take newe butter, oyle of roses, hennes grece, of eche, an ounce, put the butter and the grece, in a bygge rape roote, or i lacke of it, in a great apple, or onion & whan it is rosted softe, braye it wyth the oyle, and laye it playsterwyse vpon the kybe. ¶ An other.

Take the meate of apples and rapes rosted on the coles, of eche iii. ounces, fresh butter .ii. ounces, duckes grece or swanes grece, an ounce, stamp thē all i

Cc.ii.

The boke

a morter of lead, yf it maye be had, or els grynde them on a fayre marble & vse it

¶ Of consumption or leanesse.

When a childe cōsumeth or waxeth leane wythoute anye cause apparaūt there is a bathe commended of authours, to wasſh y chylde manye tymes, & is made thus.

Take the head and feete of a wether, seeth them tyll the bones fall a sunder, vse to bathe the chylde in this licour, & after annoynte hym wyth thys oyntement folowynge.

Take butter wythoute salte, oyle of roses and of vyolettes, of eche. i. ounce the fatte of rawe porke, halfe an ounce, waxe, a quarteron of an ounce, make ā oyntment wherwyth the chylde muste be rubbed euery daye twyse, thys with good fedinge shall encrease his strength by the grace of God.

¶ Of gogle eyes.

This impediment is neuer healed but ī a very yonge chylde, euen at y begynninge, wherevnto there is appointed

of chyldren.

ted no manner kynde of medicine, but onely an order of keppnge, that is to saye, to laye ye chylde so in hys cradelle, ye he maye beholde directe agaynste the lyght, & not to turne hys eyes on either of both sydes. If yet he begine to gogle than set ye cradell after such a fourme, that ye lyght may be on ye contrary syde, ye is on the same syde from whence he turneth hys eyes, so that for desyre of lighte he maye dyrecte them to the same part, & so by custome, bringe them to ye due fashion, and i ye nyght there ought to be a candell set in lykewyse to cause hym to behold vpon it, and remoue his eyes from the euel custome. Also grene clothes, yelowe, or purple, are verye good in thys case to be set, as is sayde afore. Furthermore a coyfe or a bygger stondyng out besydes hys eyes, to constrayne the syght to beholde direct forwarde. ❡ Of lyce.

Somtimes not only chyldren but also other ages, are annoyed with lyce, they proced of a corrupte humour, & are

engendred

engendred wythin the skynne, crepyng out a lyue thorough the poores, whiche yf they beginne to swarme in excedyng numbre, that dyseace is called of the grekes Phthiryasys, whereof Herode dyed, as is wrytten in the actes of apostles, and among the Romaynes Scilla, whych was a great tyraunt, & many other haue ben eaten of lyce to deathe, whyche thynge, whan it happeneth of the plage of God, it is paste remedye, but yf it procedeth of a naturall cause, ye maye well cure it by the meanes folowynge.

Fyrste let the paciente abstayne from all kynde of corrupte meates, or y᷑ brede scume, and emonge other, fygges and dates muste in thys case be vtterly abhorred. Than make a lauatory to wash and scoure the bodie twyse a day, thus. Take water of the sea, or els bryne and strongelye of asshes, of eche a lyke portion, wormewood a handful, seth them a whyle, and after wasshe the bodye w᷑ the same licour.

A good

of chyldren.

¶ A goodlye medicine for to kylle lyce.

Take the groūdes or dregges of oyle, aloes, wormewood, and the galle of a bulle, or of an oxe, make an oyntement whyche is singuler good for the same pourpose. ¶ An other.

Take musterde, and dissolue it in vinegre, wyth a lytle salte peter, and annoynt the places, where as the lyce are wonte to bred.

Item an herbe at the pothecaries called stauesacre, brymstone, and vynegre, is excedyng good.

It is good to gyue the pacient often in hys drynke, pouder of an hartes horne brent &c.

Stauesacre wyth oyle is a marueylouse holsom thynge in this case.

¶ An experte medicine to dryue awaye lyse.

Take the groūdes or dregges of oyle or in lack of it, fresh swines grece, a sufficient quātitie, wherin ye shal chafe an oūce of quyckspluer tyl it be all sonken into

The boke

into the grece, than take pouder of sta=
uisacre serced, and myngle all togyther,
make a gyrdyll of a wollen liste meete
for the myddle of the patient & al to an=
noynte it ouer wyth the sayde medicine
than let hym were it contynually nexte
his skinne, for it is a synguler remedi to
chase awaye the vermyn. The onely o=
dour of quyckesyluer kylleth lyce.

These shal be suffycient to declare at
this tyme in this litle treatise of ye cure
of chyldren which yf I maye knowe to
be thankefully receyued I wil by gods
grace supplye more hereafter, neyther
desyre I any lenger to lyue than I wil
employe my studyes to the honoure of
god, and profyt of the weale publike.

⁋ Thus endeth ye booke of childerne
composed by Thomas
Phayer, studiouse
in Philosophie
and Phisicke.

The Table.

¶ The contentes of the regiment of lyfe.

Of diseases & remedyes of ye heed.
Payne commyng of choler,
Payne caused of fleume,
Payne caused of melancholye,
Regiment for all heedache.
Remedye for heedache of all causes.
Of diseases in the face.
To pallifye a face vncurable
For rednesse of the face.
For cankers, vlcers, and Noli me tangere.
For wormes in the face,
A purgation for the same,
Dyete for the same syckneffe
For the eyes, and to quycken ye sight.
For payne in the eyes.
For bloodshotten eyes.
For swellyng of the eyes,
For sore eyes.
For great payne in the eyes,
For rednesse in the eyes.
For hardnesse in the eyes,

For

The table.

For all rednesse of eyes.
To dye the eyes.
For webbes in the eyes.
Regiment for diseases in the eyes.
For infirmities of the eares.
For stynkyng of the nose.
For nosebleadyng.
Remedye for tothache.
To make teeth whyte.
Remedyes for diseases in the brest.
For a horse voyce.
For the cough.
For shortnesse of wynde.
For asthma.
An oyntment for the breath.
Regiment for the same.
Remedies for phthysyke.
For the pleuresye.
For diseases in the rybbes.
Weakenesse of the hert and the cure.
Swownyng.
For diseases of the stomake.
For weaknes therof.
For abhorryng of meate.
For belchyng.

For

The table.

For wyndynesse thereof.
For the hycket,
Regiment for hycket.
For vomytyng.
To comfort the stomake.
Peyne in the stomake.
Remedyes for diseases of þ lyuer.
A singuler purgatiō for cholere.
Other medicines laxatyue.
For heate in the liuer.
For stoppyng of the liuer.
Remedye for diseases of the galle.
For Jaundyes.
For diseases in the splene.
A goodly purgation for melācholy.
For the blacke Jaundys.
For all oppilations.
Diseases of the bowels.
For colyke and yliaca passio.
For the wyndye colyke.
A suppositorye,

A purgation

The table.

A purgation for collyke of fleume.
A glystre for all colyke.
Payne of the reynes, and remedye.
Dyete for colyke and peyne of the reynes.
Fluxes of the bellye.
Remedye for the fluxe lienteria.
For the fluxe dyarhea and other.
Lectuaries for the fluxe.
For fluxe of all causes.
Diseases of the matryce.
To staunche the fluxe of women.
For stranglyng of the matrice.
For al paynes of the mother.
Of the stone in the reynes and bladder, wyth the perfyte cure and dyete for the same.
Of the goute, wyth the causes and remedyes.

¶ Finis.

The

The table.
¶ The contentes of the treatyse of the pestilence.

In the fyrste parte.
A preface of the author.
What is signifyed by thys woorde pestilence.
The firste rote or cause superior of the pestilence.
The seconde rote superior.
The thyrde roote, inferiour.
The fourth rote, or cause interior.
Of election of the ayer.
Of eatynge and drynkynge.
Of slepyng and wakyng.
Of excercyse.
Of emptines and fulnes.
Of accidentes of the mynde.
Of medicines preseruatyues.
A drynke for the pestilence.
A good preseruatiue for ye comō people
A pouder for the same.
An other siguler remedye for riche mē.
An other soueraygne and goodly receit
bothe

The table.

bothe preseruatyue and curatiue.
Of swete waters.
Perfumes agaynst the pestilence.
Pomaunders for pestylence.
  In the seconde parte.
How to knowe a person infected.
Of the cure of pestilence by the way of diete.
Of the cure of pestilence by the way of medicines.
A recept agaynst the pestilence.
Manardus medicine,
Alectuary of great vertue.
An other medicine liquyde.
Of lettyng blood, vētoses & purgatiōs
Of application of outward medicines
A playstre to rype a botche cōmynge of the pestilence.
An other for the same.
The vse of surgerye for hym that hath no botche.
Of the cure of carbuncles and anthrax.
A good defensyue.
A declaracion of the vtilitie of veynes cōmonly to be let blood in the bodye of man.   Finis.

¶ Imprinted at london in Fletestrete at the signe of the Sunne ouer against the conduyte, by Edward Whitchurche the last daye of June.

1.5.4.6.

¶ Cum priuilegio ad imprimendum solum.